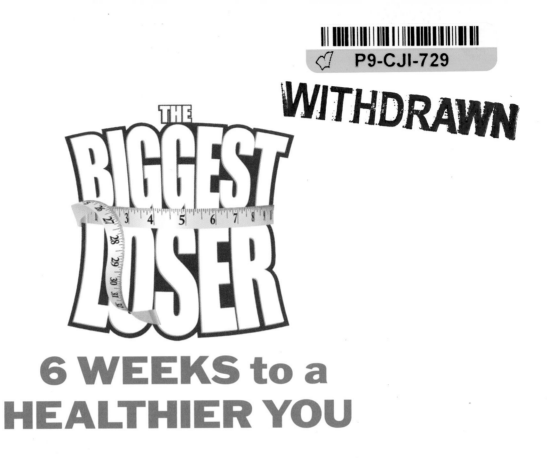

THE BIGGEST LOSER

6 WEEKS to a HEALTHIER YOU

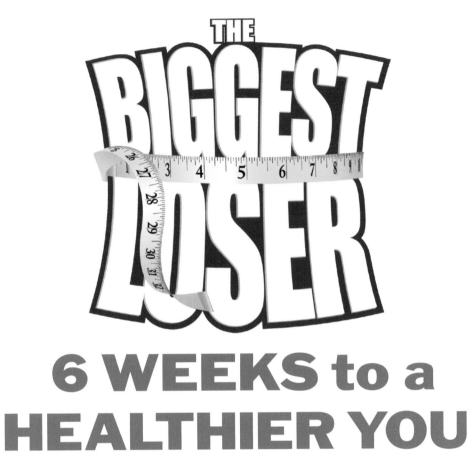

6 WEEKS to a HEALTHIER YOU

Lose Weight and Get Healthy for Life!

Cheryl Forberg, RD, Melissa Roberson, Lisa Wheeler,
and *The Biggest Loser* Experts and Cast

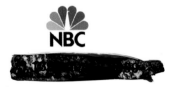

© 2010 by Universal City Studios Productions LLLP, Inc. The Biggest Loser is a registered trademark and copyright of NBC Studios, Inc., and Reveille LLC. Licensed by NBC Universal Television Consumer Products Group. All rights reserved.

All rights reserved. No part of this publication may be reproduced or transmitted in any form or by any means, electronic or mechanical, including photocopying, recording, or any other information storage and retrieval system, without the written permission of the publisher.

Rodale books may be purchased for business or promotional use or for special sales. For information, please write to: Special Markets Department, Rodale Inc., 733 Third Avenue, New York, NY 10017.

Printed in the United States of America
Rodale Inc. makes every effort to use acid-free ♾, recycled paper ♲.

Book design by Christina Gaugler
Illustration on page 32 by Judy Newhouse
Recipe photographs by Mitch Mandel/Rodale Images. Food styling by Diane Vezza and prop styling by Pamela Simpson.
Exercise photographs by Thomas McDonald/Rodale Images. Hair and makeup by Adrienne Bearden and clothing by Inessah Selditz.
All other photos by NBC Universal Photo.

Library of Congress Cataloging-in-Publication Data

Forberg, Cheryl.
   The biggest loser. 6 weeks to a healthier you : lose weight and get healthy for life! / Cheryl Forberg, Melissa Roberson, Lisa Wheeler ; and The Biggest Loser Experts and Cast.
      p.   cm.
   Includes index.
   ISBN-13 978-1-60529-514-5 pbk.
   ISBN-10 1-60529-514-0 pbk.
   1. Obesity—Complications—Prevention—Popular works. 2. Weight loss—Popular works. I. Roberson, Melissa. II. Wheeler, Lisa. III. Biggest loser (Television program). IV. Title.
RC628.F667 2010
613.2'5—dc22
                                        2010000154

Distributed to the trade by Macmillan
2 4 6 8 10 9 7 5 3 1   paperback

REVEILLE

We inspire and enable people to improve their lives and the world around them
For more of our products visit **rodalestore.com** or call 800-848-4735

Production Development & Direction: Chad Bennett, Dave Broome, Neysa Gordon, Mark Koops, Kim Niemi, Todd Nelson, J. D. Roth, and Ben Silverman

NBCU, Reveille, 25/7 Productions, and 3Ball Productions would like to thank the many people who gave their time and energy to this project:

Jenna Alifante, Stephen Andrade, Carole Angelo, Dana Arnett, Sebastian Attie, Nancy N. Bailey, Dave Bjerke, Maria Bohe, Jill Bowles, *The Biggest Loser* contestants, Joni Camacho, Jill Carmen, Scot Chastain, Hope Clarke, Ben Cohen, Jason Cooper, Steve Coulter, Marie Crousillat, Dan Curran, Dr. Michael Dansinger, Jenny Ellis, Kat Elmore, Sione Fa, John Farrell, Cheryl Forberg, Joseph Ford, Devin Franchino, Jeff Friedman, Jeff Gaspin, Christina Gaugler, Marc Graboff, Bob Harper, Chris Harris, Julie Ann Harris, Robyn Hennessey, Shelli Hill, Dr. Robert Huizenga, Matthew Jacobs, Jill Jarosz, Helen Jorda, Adam Kaloustian, Alex Katz, Allison Kaz, Loretta Kraft, Chris Krogermeier, Laura Kuhn, Beth Lamb, Todd Lubin, Roni Lubliner, Alan Lundgren, Carole MacDonal, Rebecca Marks, Joaquin Mesa, Jillian Michaels, Gregg Michaelson, Lily Milkovic-Jakal, John Miller, Ann Morteo, Kam Naderi, Gabriela Navarro, Julie Nugent, Trae Patton, Jerry Petry, Helen Phillips, Ellie Prezant, Ed Prince, Lee Rierson, Karen Rinaldi, Melissa Roberson, Beth Roberts, Maria Rodale, Jessica Roth, Joe Schlosser, Leslie Schwartz, Robin Shallow, Carrie Simons, Mitch Steele, Lee Straus, Kelia Tardiff, Paul Teledgy, Deborah Thomas, Julie True, Ali Vincent, Lisa Wheeler, Liza Whitcraft, Julie Will, Audrey Wood, Yong Yam, Jeff Zucker

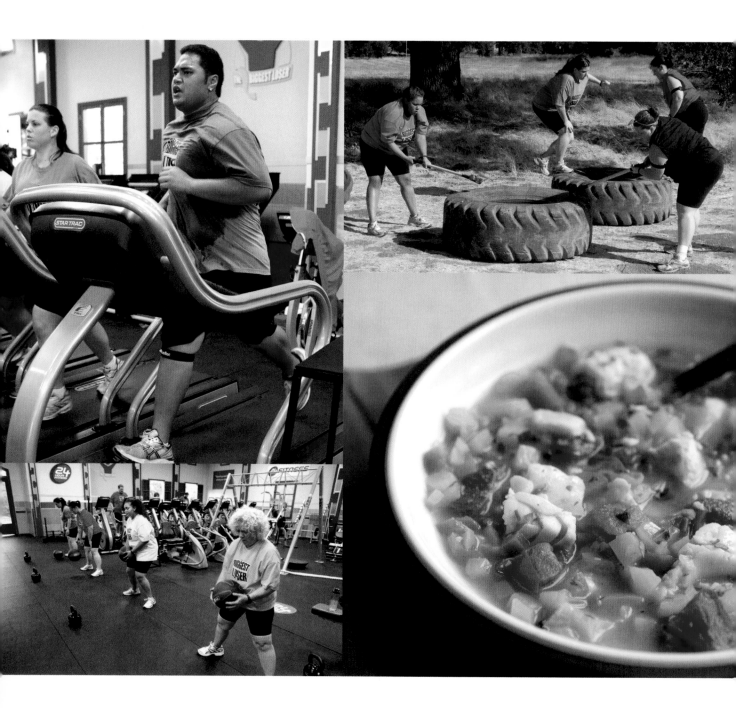

Contents

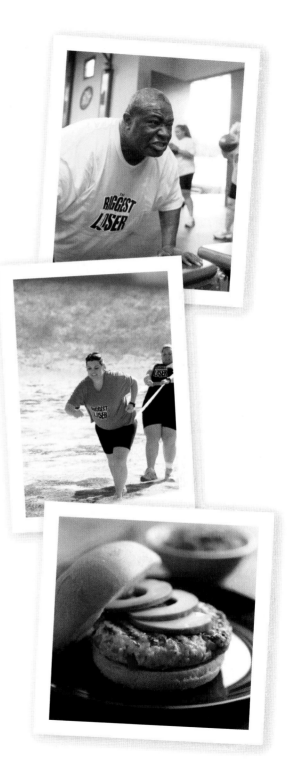

Introduction

What's at Stake

As the editor of BiggestLoserClub.com, I am in touch daily with current and former *Biggest Loser* contestants, many of whom I have known now for years. And I am in constant contact with *The Biggest Loser* team, including the trainers, Dr. Robert Huizenga, and nutritionist Cheryl Forberg, who share their advice for our online subscribers and keep me in the loop with training tips, medical advice, and new recipes. I also visit the Ranch a few times each season to get to know the contestants in person.

The day before the Season 8 finale, I took a colleague to visit *The Biggest Loser* Ranch for the first time and to meet some of the Season 9 contestants. Cheryl Forberg had just taken the group grocery shopping, and they had come back to cook lean beef, slaw, and other delicious, healthy meals. Everyone was chatting in the kitchen, the Ranch's heartbeat as it is in every home. My colleague marveled at Daris George's thick curly hair. She admired Michael Venterella's big blue eyes. She appreciated Sherry Johnston's personality. We were catching up with O'Neal Hampton when a cheer erupted. Coach Mo DeWalt from Season 8 was in the house! Ever the coach, he wanted to drop in on his way to the finale and encourage the new crop of contestants.

"When I got here, I was extremely overweight," he told them. "I was sick, I had diabetes, I couldn't walk to the gym without pain. I was 55, but my body was 70. This turned out to be the journey of my life. This is not about the show," he said. "This is about getting your health back, your life back. You're part of a family now."

As my colleague and I left the Ranch, all hugged and kissed from meeting our new friends, we felt part of a family, too. "What an amazing group of people," she said. "What great stories, what heart and soul."

It's the one thing critics of the show always get wrong. These people don't come to the Ranch for money, they come for love. Sometimes they know it's because they love someone else ("Why do you think I came to this dumb old place?" Bette-Sue Burklund tearily asked her daughter Ali Vincent during Season 5). But often it's because they fall in love with someone else—themselves.

Good health is self-love, in the end. And it's something every single contestant leaves with. Everyone wins. And they win the most important prize of all.

As one of the newest contestants, O'Neal Hampton says, "For me, the prize is my health. Not just about how many pounds I lost in a week. My new healthy lifestyle is the most important thing to me."

And from one of the first contestants, Dave Fioravanti of Season 1, "My weight loss and knowing how to live healthy makes me live in the now and keep it real. I have a whole, loving, healthy life and before the show, it was bedlam and chaos. Today, I live in complete peace."

Cheryl, Lisa, and I—and *The Biggest Loser* experts and cast—hope this book not only gives you the tools to a healthier you but also brings you the life you deserve. It's something everyone should have.

—Melissa Roberson

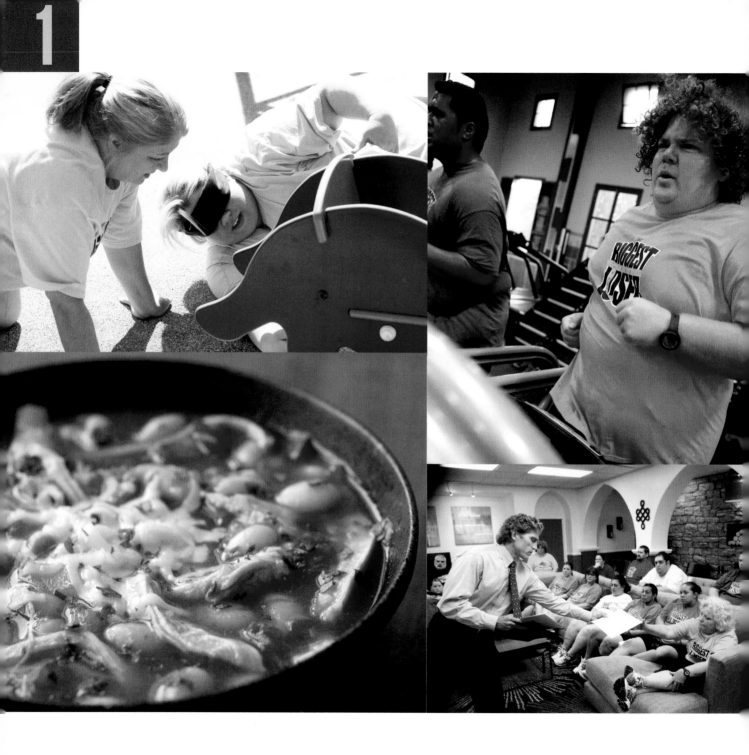

Start the Journey

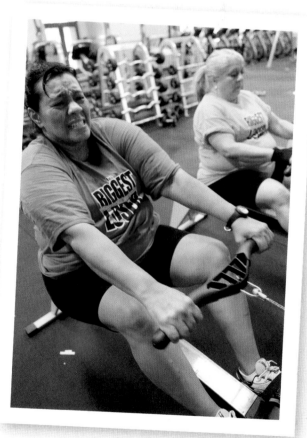

ontestants come to *The Biggest Loser* Ranch for a variety of reasons. Yes, the grand prize (and the bragging rights) provides some motivation, but every *Biggest Loser* is looking to win big in other ways. For the Season 9 contestants—the heaviest cast in *Biggest Loser* history—it's about winning back their health, their lives, and the ability to be the person they've always wanted to be.

At 403 pounds, Gray Team member Koli Palu says he knew he needed to change his life because "death is at my doorstep; it really is." Lance Morgan, the 365-pound Texas rancher, says he felt he had two options: Get healthy or end up in "a pine box." For twins James and John Crutchfield, weighing in at 485 and 484 pounds respectively, coming to *The Biggest Loser* Ranch was about not becoming another statistic in a family that has seen numerous members suffer from obesity-related health issues such as diabetes, stroke, and gastric bypass surgery.

As the title suggests, this book is about reclaiming health—and *you!* Since the end of Season 8, more than 18,200 pounds have been lost by contestants on *The Biggest Loser.* And when they shed all that extra weight, they also shed things like blood pressure medication, type 2 diabetes, depression, and all the inhibitions that have kept them from living their fullest, best lives—both mentally and physically.

Twenty-five-year-old Daris George, who came to the Ranch for Season 9 with his mom, Cheryl, says that taking off his shirt and showing the world what he had become was one of the scariest things he'd ever done. Change is never easy, especially when you don't recognize yourself in the mirror. But every season on *The Biggest Loser,* we watch as the contestants fight hard to take back ownership of their lives. And once they get a taste of what it's like to feel healthy, happy, and just plain good—they never want to revert back to their old habits. As Season 9's Maria Ventrella says, "Overcoming your fears is so important. If you don't overcome them, you'll just bring them about in a different way."

Brown Team

James Crutchfield

AGE: 30
STARTING WEIGHT: 485 pounds
HEIGHT: 6'5"
HOMETOWN: Orlando, Florida

John Crutchfield

AGE: 30
STARTING WEIGHT: 484 pounds
HEIGHT: 6'5"
HOMETOWN: Orlando, Florida

With a combined weight of almost 1,000 pounds, the Crutchfield brothers nicknamed themselves the "half-ton twins." Brown Team members James and John have been overweight since they were 10 years old. Amazingly, they've always been within a few pounds of each other. Though they played sports in high school, now that they've turned 30 and their weight has reached an all-time high, the twins are no longer able to participate in activities they once enjoyed.

Before he arrived at the Ranch, James landed in the hospital with soaring high blood pressure. He could no longer go dancing with his wife or even take long walks. "This isn't how I wanted the world to see me," he says.

John, who has a 1-year-old son, worries about his family's history of diabetes and obesity. Recent deaths in the family haunt him. "My dad died, then 2 months later my grandma, then a sister, then a friend. My mom had a mild stroke and is overweight and wheelchair bound. I felt cursed and turned to food for comfort." The first word spoken by his baby boy was "Da-da," and John refuses to leave his son fatherless.

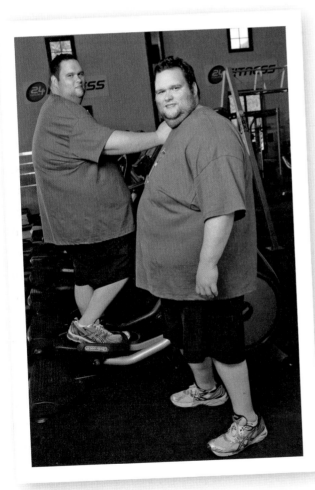

The twins say they no longer want to use food as a source of comfort. And after arriving at *The Biggest Loser* Ranch and embarking on a healthy new lifestyle, they're turning things around.

Today, James says he feels much better. "I am active and go to the gym every single day. I am capable of so much more than I expected. My life has been made better because I realize I can do this. I know what to do. I have all the tools to succeed and live a long, healthy life with my wife. This whole process has brought my wife and me closer."

The twins can now swim and bike long distances and are more positive about their future. "I've gained an understanding of my body and its capabilities," says John. "Eating all that healthy food, it really makes a difference! I have a lot more energy and am more positive and excited for the future. I've gained a new lease on life."

The two continue to push each other to get healthy and to make sure their health causes no further family heartache.

Red Team

Melissa Morgan

AGE: 39

STARTING WEIGHT: 233 pounds

HEIGHT: 5'6"

HOMETOWN: Aspermont, Texas

Lance Morgan

AGE: 37

STARTING WEIGHT: 365 pounds

HEIGHT: 6'3"

HOMETOWN: Aspermont, Texas

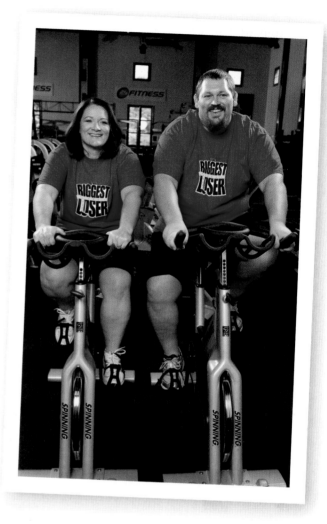

Melissa and Lance Morgan are the first to admit that weight has taken a toll on their marriage. "We made a commitment to each other 10 years ago. We need to go back to who we were then, because we're just not there anymore. Our weight is seriously affecting us as a couple," they admit. "We're really at a point where we say things like 'Shut up, don't talk to me.' We don't have respect for each other."

Lance admits that before they arrived at the Ranch, "it had gotten to the point that all we did at home was eat and bicker."

Melissa packed on 40 pounds in the early years of their marriage and added another 20 after the birth of her children. While she was busy with law school, the family ate takeout. For Lance, his weight cost him his job as a professional scuba diver when he could no longer pass the required physical. "We can't afford to sit back and pretend that our weight is not an issue," says Melissa. "I'm an attorney. I have to project confidence in front of a jury. And I feel like a moose in the courtroom."

Now that they've embarked on their weight-loss journey together, "it's about forever," says Melissa. "It's not so much about the game as it is about health and fitness. This is an emotional and psychological change for me. I'm an emotional eater. And I know that food doesn't fix anything."

Today, the benefits of weight loss are rolling in. "I feel so much better," says Lance. "My feet don't hurt all the time, I can walk for more than 30 minutes, and I can breathe! I am looking forward to getting out and doing things with my kids instead of just sitting around the house with them."

"We made a commitment to our community," Melissa remarks about their weight-loss goals. "We have a huge amount of support back home. We want to bring back what we learn here and get it out to our community in Texas. We want people to understand that you don't need to eat a 44-ounce anything."

Reflecting on her new level of fitness, Melissa says, "Before I came to the Ranch, I refused to push through to the next level. Today, I know that I have the ability to push through. It's really mind over matter. You just have to find your drive and desire."

Melissa Morgan, Season 9

Health and fitness were my main reasons for being on *The Biggest Loser*. Today, my blood pressure is under control without medication. I can climb stairs or walk a mile without being completely out of breath. I'm going to be 40 in February, and I want my next 40 years to be full of life.

Purple Team

Patti Anderson

AGE: 55

STARTING WEIGHT: 243 pounds

HEIGHT: 5'4"

HOMETOWN: Lafayette, California

Stephanie Anderson

AGE: 29

STARTING WEIGHT: 264 pounds

HEIGHT: 5'8"

HOMETOWN: West Hollywood, California

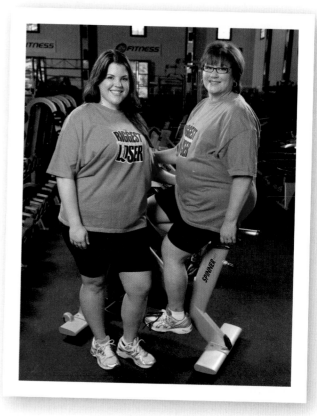

Patti Anderson has the dubious distinction of having about the worst case of diabetes that *The Biggest Loser* medical expert Dr. Robert Huizenga has ever seen. She arrived at the Ranch on nine medications, and teammate and daughter Stephanie was quickly following in her mother's footsteps. Based on her *Biggest Loser* Know Your Number Healthscore, Dr. Huizenga predicted that Stephanie would develop the disease before she turned 36.

Patti battled being overweight as a child and lost her dad suddenly when he turned 55. Today, she wants to enjoy as many healthy years with her family as possible. She truly understands now what Dr. Huizenga told her the first week on the Ranch: Type 2 diabetes is reversible through diet and exer-

cise. "It made me incredibly sad to see what we had done to ourselves," Patti laments.

For Stephanie, the challenge will be finding a balance between taking care of herself and being in a high-pressure job. "I'm going to find ongoing motivation in my friends and family who believe in me," she says. "Those are people who want me to succeed and who support me every step of the way."

Stephanie already feels more energetic now that the weight is coming off. "Mom told me not to limit myself. And I'm not going to."

Gray Team

Sam Poueu

AGE: **23**

STARTING WEIGHT: **372 pounds**

HEIGHT: **6'4"**

HOMETOWN: **Rohnert Park, California**

Koli Palu

AGE: **28**

STARTING WEIGHT: **403 pounds**

HEIGHT: **6'1"**

HOMETOWN: **Rohnert Park, California**

Koli Palu and Sam Poueu were inspired by the successful weight loss of another pair of Tongan cousins—Season 7's Sione and Filipe Fa. Coming from a culture rife with obesity-related diseases, Sam and Koli know they have their work cut out for them.

"I'm going to sit down with my family and have a long talk about nutrition, the kind of food we should eat, and the 50-pound bags of rice in the house," says Sam. He and Koli work as bouncers at night and Koli says, "We'd grab the quickest thing on the way to work. I never thought about what I put in my mouth. Now I'm weighing everything and counting calories."

The Gray Team cousins coach football, and Koli says he used to put his team through some hard workouts that he couldn't do himself. That's all changing. "As a coach, I know our bodies are amazing things," says Koli. "I need my football team to understand that you can go that extra step. This is more of a mental game, a mental toughness. As long as you push yourself, the physical part will be there."

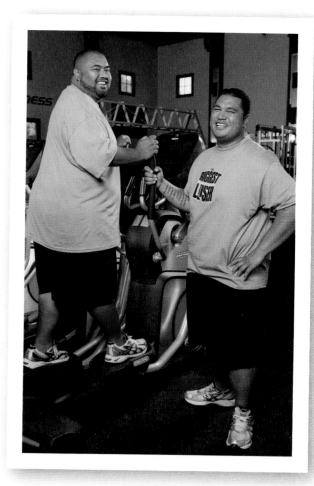

Black Team

Darrell Hough

AGE: 46

STARTING WEIGHT: 413 pounds

HEIGHT: 5'10"

HOMETOWN: Ann Arbor, Michigan

Andrea Hough

AGE: 24

STARTING WEIGHT: 298 pounds

HEIGHT: 5'7"

HOMETOWN: Ann Arbor, Michigan

"I did more in my first 3 days on the Ranch than I'd done in 20 years, and I'm still alive," laughs Darrell Hough.

"It was an intense first workout," adds daughter and teammate Andrea. "Every muscle in my body was crying out. I was an athlete growing up. I played sports in high school. That's what saved me from gaining weight. But after that, the weight piled on. I'd forgotten what it's like to be an athlete. I'm excited to get that back."

Darrell remembers being an overweight kid who wore "husky"-size jeans. "I had to roll them up—they were for someone taller," he says. "In junior high, I weighed in the 200s. In high school, I was well into the 300s. Obesity runs in my family. But in my family, I felt totally loved and accepted. It was outside the family where I got teased. I played sports but always got picked last because I was the slowest."

"He's been overweight my whole life," says Andrea of her father. "It's never hindered my love for him, but I want him to be healthy. *I* want to be healthy. I want us to get healthy together. So this is a dream come true. He's realizing he's able to do it. He got in the pool the other day for the first time in 20 years. He hadn't wanted to wear a swimsuit in public."

"Through workouts, I'm finding my problem is mental," says Darrell. "My fear of what's going to happen has been dictating my participation in everything. If someone wanted to go canoeing, I would be afraid my back would hurt. I'm excited to stop that cycle.

"You need to take fitness and weight loss as seriously as you would take your job," he says.

"Make it part of what you do every day. Apply yourself. Learn what to do and measure your job performance in terms of weight loss, which, in turn, will keep you motivated.

"Keep in mind that the more weight you lose," he adds, "the more energy you'll have for working out. Even my joints feel better now that the pounds are coming off. When you get tired or discouraged, remember that's only momentary. Losing weight is going to give you a positive outlook for the rest of your life."

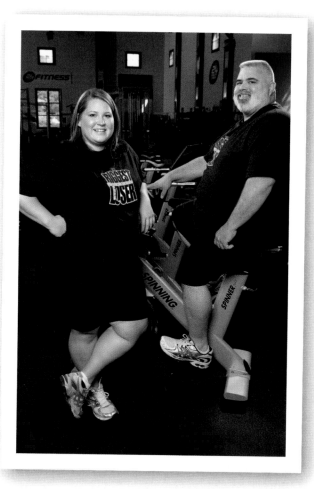

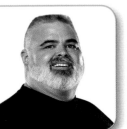

Darrell Hough, Season 9

I now love salad mixed with veggies. I have one at almost every meal, because it provides lots of bulk with few calories.

Green Team

Miggy Cancel

AGE: 47

STARTING WEIGHT: 240 pounds

HEIGHT: 5'9"

HOMETOWN: Pemberton, New Jersey

Migdalia Sebren

AGE: 28

STARTING WEIGHT: 265 pounds

HEIGHT: 5'9"

HOMETOWN: Sanford, North Carolina

Coming from a Puerto Rican culture, mother and daughter Miggy and Migdalia realize their eating habits have a lot to do with their weight gain. "There was always something frying in our kitchen," says Miggy. "At a family reunion, I found out a lot of family members were sick with diabetes, one brother had a stroke, another a heart attack. And everyone sort of said, 'Well, you're next, these diseases are in the family genes.' Someone has to change these genes. It was a wake-up call."

Today, Miggy and Migdalia are setting small goals every day. "I'm walking/running 2 miles a day every day," says Miggy. "That adds up to 14 miles in a week, a little more than a half-marathon.

I used to be afraid to swim, but I've overcome that and plan to keep swimming at least once a week and build up to more as time goes by."

Migdalia is motivated to keep herself healthy for her young children. With a husband bound for a tour of duty in Afghanistan, she knows how much they depend on her. Her mother stays motivated by looking back at her hard work and how it's already adding up. "How is my life different since losing weight?" she muses. "Well, I can now bend over to tie my shoes without getting short of breath. I'm off my meds and am saving money on prescriptions. I'm able to move and think and analyze things from a different perspective—a calmer, easier, less overwhelmed perspective."

Their new rallying cry for weight loss? *¡Sí, se puede!* "Yes, we can!"

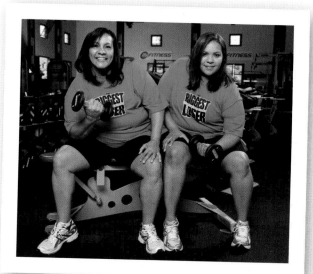

Orange Team

Cheryl George

AGE: 50

STARTING WEIGHT: 227 pounds

HEIGHT: 5'4"

HOMETOWN: Ardmore, Oklahoma

Daris George

AGE: 25

STARTING WEIGHT: 346 pounds

HEIGHT: 5'10"

HOMETOWN: Ardmore, Oklahoma

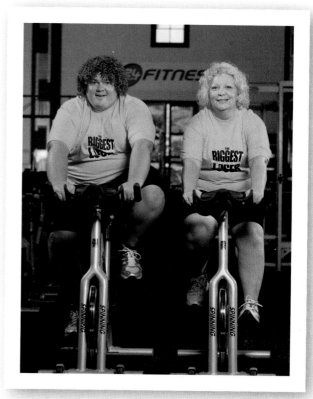

"It's not about the money," says Daris of his motivation to try out for *The Biggest Loser,* "it's about what you can do. In the first few weeks at the Ranch, I experienced things I'd never done in my life."

Teammate and mom Cheryl agrees: "I spent more time on the treadmill in my first week at the Ranch than I've spent on a treadmill in my entire life!"

Daris lives at home with his parents, but his mom wants to see him have the kind of life a young man deserves. She knows he feels protective of her, since her husband frequently travels for business. Already, she's discovered that Daris's confidence is building. "My smile is getting bigger every day," he agrees.

What's the first thing he wants to do when he resumes his new life at home? "I'm going to ask someone on a date. I've never done that before. In social situations, I'm a fun person, but I'm also the person who goes home alone."

"We know we're both our own people, that we're here for each other but also for ourselves," says Cheryl. "I know what a big heart he has. Whoever that first date is, Mom's going to be close behind thinking, 'You'd better be here for the right reasons.'"

White Team

Maria Ventrella

AGE: 51

STARTING WEIGHT: 281 pounds

HEIGHT: 5'4"

HOMETOWN: Chicago, Illinois

Michael Ventrella

AGE: 30

STARTING WEIGHT: 526 pounds

HEIGHT: 6'3"

HOMETOWN: Chicago, Illinois

White Team member Michael Ventrella is the heaviest person ever to walk onto *The Biggest Loser* campus. But after just a few days at the Ranch, Michael and his mom, Maria, were already feeling the effects of a new life. "My underwear is loose!" exults Michael. "I'm holding up my pants with a belt!" chimes in Maria.

"I feel so alive. I'm eating right. I'm working out. I'm sleeping. If you get all three of those components, you're going to succeed," says Michael. This is a big change from his life as a deejay, in which he usually grabbed fast food on the way home from work. He called his eating life "a constant consumption of horrible things."

Now he thinks about his hunger—is it in his head or truly in his gut?

The mother/son team felt tested in the 26.2-mile bike challenge. "I thought, you know, this is TV," says Michael. "They'll put us on the bikes for a few minutes and then go to a commercial break. Nope. I've never seen anyone throw up that much in my life," he adds, pointing to his mom.

"Before I came to the Ranch," says Maria, "I didn't walk at all. I didn't even walk to the mailbox. I'm a shy person. I've been afraid to do a lot of things. But I'm not going to be afraid anymore. I can walk on a treadmill. I can ride a bike. I had never biked in my life! I grew up in a traditional Italian house where women cleaned and cooked. I didn't go outside. I got married, had kids. I cleaned and cooked, I went to work. That was my life. After this? Hey, everybody for themselves! I want to live! I want to run in 5-Ks! I've lost so much time, and I want a different life."

"I'm so proud of my mother," says Michael. "I've seen her do things that I never could have fathomed. On the treadmill yesterday, she was like a cheetah! She went for 50 minutes—and I was struggling with 20.

"For so long, my weight has owned my happiness," admits Michael. "It's dominated every facet of my life. If friends invite me to a picnic, I worry ahead of time: What am I going to wear? Where can I sit? Are people going to stare at me? It's easier to just stay at home.

"I want to meet the woman of my dreams. I want to get married and have a family," says Michael. "It's not going to happen looking and feeling this way. I feel like if I can't love myself, no one else will love me. Never in my worst nightmares did I think that I'd be this big. Even if I lose 200 pounds, I'll still be overweight. But I've been emotional about my weight for way too long. It's time to fight this battle. I want to do this now, because I'm saving my life."

Most important, he says, "I came to this journey with an open heart. I'm ready."

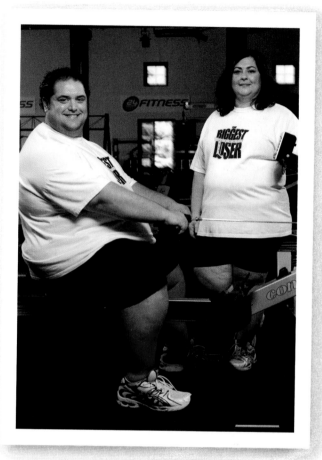

Michael Ventrella, Season 9

Plan a daily routine that's going to work for *you* and *your* lifestyle. For me, one of the greatest workout machines is the stair climber. Not so long ago, at 526 pounds, I would not be able to do 5 minutes on that thing. But now I am working out on a daily average of 90 minutes or more.

Yellow Team

O'Neal Hampton

AGE: 50

STARTING WEIGHT: 389 pounds

HEIGHT: 5'11"

HOMETOWN: Minneapolis, Minnesota

SunShine Hampton

AGE: 23

STARTING WEIGHT: 275 pounds

HEIGHT: 5'6"

HOMETOWN: Minneapolis, Minnesota

Losing a brother who was only 58 finally made Yellow Team member O'Neal Hampton realize that life is precious and fleeting. Now he and daughter SunShine are on their way to healthier living. "I feel emancipated," says O'Neal. "I'm finally getting rid of this weight."

Both father and daughter are former athletes. O'Neal played football. SunShine was a synchronized swimmer in high school, but says it's been a long time since she's worn a bathing suit. "It breaks my heart, because I love to swim," she says. "I want to get a bikini!"

"I want her to lose weight for every reason except that one!" responds the ever-protective father.

Finding himself close to 400 pounds, O'Neal scoffed at people who tried to reassure him by saying that he was "big boned." "That's just lying," he says. "That's worse than being teased."

He goes by the nickname "Big O'Neal," but the name has more to do with the size of his spirit than his body. There are 18 inches, he says, from your heart to your head. If you can connect those two, nothing can stop you. "I hadn't made that connection," O'Neal says. "Now I have."

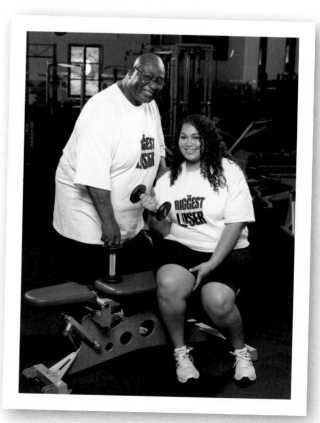

Blue Team

Cherita Andrews

AGE: 50

STARTING WEIGHT: 277 pounds

HEIGHT: 5'8"

HOMETOWN: Houston, Texas

Vicky Andrews

AGE: 22

STARTING WEIGHT: 358 pounds

HEIGHT: 5'9"

HOMETOWN: Houston, Texas

If you watched the first episode of Season 9, you saw that mother/daughter team Cherita and Vicky Andrews faced their worst nightmare: They were eliminated in the very first challenge and sent home for 30 days.

"We were devastated," says Cherita. "We had built up so much hope about what we'd learn on the Ranch—and then we were sent home."

But they returned home armed with advice from trainers Bob Harper and Jillian Michaels, as well as the guidelines of *The Biggest Loser* eating plan. They had 30 days to work out and eat right at home before competing to win their spot back on the Ranch. Cherita and Vicky were determined to make it back.

"After I got over the devastation of being elimi-

nated," says Cherita, "I thought, 'You know what? I'm one of those bottom-line kind of girls.' We had already made the decision to lose the weight. We stood before family and friends and said, 'Failure is not an option.' Did we mean that?"

The Blue Team members say they draw their inspiration and motivation from friends and family members. After they told the people in their lives that they would get healthy, they felt responsible for putting action behind their words.

"It's about doing your best," adds Vicky. "We'll get there."

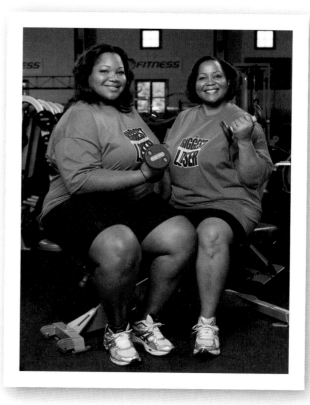

Pink Team

Sherry Johnston

AGE: 51

STARTING WEIGHT: 218 pounds

HEIGHT: 5'1"

HOMETOWN: Knoxville, Tennessee

Ashley Johnston

AGE: 27

STARTING WEIGHT: 374 pounds

HEIGHT: 5'5"

HOMETOWN: Knoxville, Tennessee

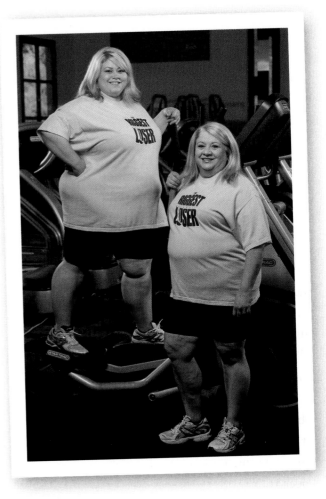

It's a funny thing about deciding to get healthy. You might be motivated to change your life for somebody else, but you can't be successful unless you're also doing it for yourself. Pink Team member Sherry Johnston says, "I thought I was coming here for my daughter. But I realized I came for me." And that was after trying to bribe everyone they knew to join daughter Ashley at the Ranch. "I tried to convince other family members to come with her—I was supposed to be the backup, and here I am!"

Sherry has been a single mom since her husband died of cancer 11 years ago, and that's when she turned to food for comfort. She's been leading a grief support group and working for a nonprofit organization. But she wasn't taking care of herself physically. "It's like when you fly, and they tell you that in case of an emergency, you need to put on your oxygen mask first before you can help someone else. Well, that's what I'm doing.

"Now that I'm seeing changes in my body as I lose weight, it motivates me to do more and to keep going," Sherry says. "And it all started with a little movement! I know the weight loss is helping me to be better. I am working hard, and I'm going to live longer for it. The doctor reports are getting better as I lose more weight."

It's the small celebrations she loves. "I sat down the other day and, look at that, I crossed my legs! It's been a long time since I've been able to do that."

By the time Ashley was in high school, she wore a size 14 or 16 and continued to gain, putting on more than 100 pounds. "I hated to run into old friends and classmates because I felt embarrassed about my weight. I felt stuck in a body that did not allow me to live life, to be myself—to dress in the kind of clothes I like!"

Like others on the Ranch, Ashley discovered that she enjoys running, and she plans to continue it at home. "A runner once told me that it's great to run in the morning while the world is sleeping, because you get to see things that you normally wouldn't. I was always so tired before. I had severe sleep apnea and found out that I wasn't getting restful sleep. Now I have more energy than ever. And I love to sweat! I never wanted to push myself

to that point before. Now I find that the more I sweat, the better, I feel.

"I have never lost weight, only gained. To be able to get rid of old clothes because they're too large is an amazing feeling. I definitely feel more confident, secure, sexy, and just more like who I knew I was on the inside. My health is so much better, and my goals seem achievable and reachable. I feel amazing."

Sherry Johnston, Season 9

I used to be intimidated by all the equipment in the gym. But get a trainer to show you how to use just a couple of machines. Most gyms have someone on the floor who knows how things work. That's why they're there, to help you. Ask for help!

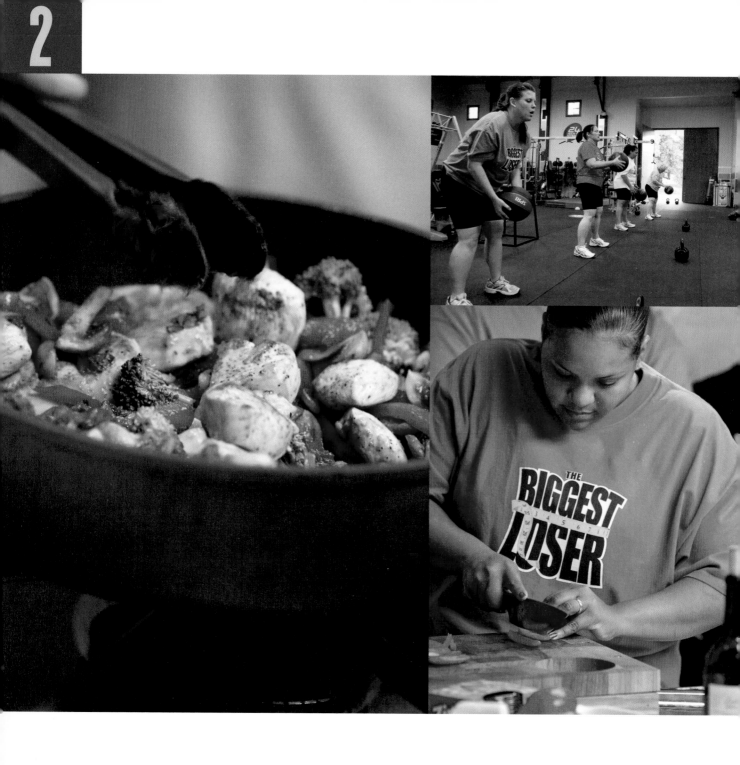

2

Eat for Optimum Health

On the day contestants first arrive at *The Biggest Loser* Ranch, nutritionist Cheryl Forberg meets with them for some nutrition boot camp—they shop, cook, study *The Biggest Loser* books, and learn to master healthy new recipes. The former fast-food junkies soon become experts in counting calories and measuring portion sizes. By the second week on the ranch, you'll hear contestants confidently saying, "There are 150 calories in this cup of turkey chili. I think I'll have it as part of my 300-calorie lunch."

Cheryl gives the contestants a crash course in good nutrition as well as in the fundamentals of eating for weight loss—which includes paying close attention to portions, measuring and weighing food, tracking calories through a food journal, and aiming to get the most nutrient-dense or "good" calories into each day as possible.

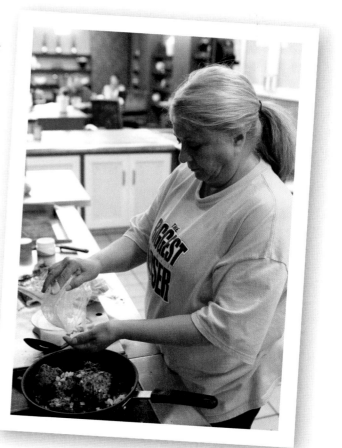

Calorie Budgets

In calculating calories for weight loss, some formulas can get pretty elaborate, requiring a lot of math. Although the calorie budgets for *The Biggest Loser* contestants at the Ranch are based on comprehensive body composition calculations as well as metabolic testing, here's a rule of thumb for people at home: Most people need a daily caloric range of somewhere between 7 and 10 calories per pound for long-term weight-loss success, or a minimum of 1,200 calories per day.

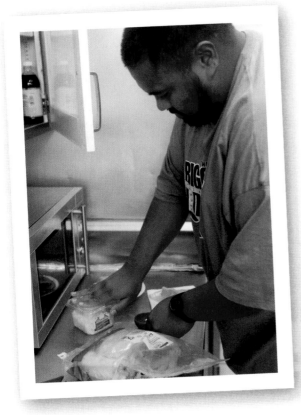

Keep in mind, though, that everyone is unique in the way they lose weight, and we all burn different numbers of calories at different rates. So if you and a partner, friend, or buddy follow *The Biggest Loser* eating plan, one person might lose weight at a different rate—faster or slower—from week to week. Just like the contestants on *The Biggest Loser,* you may drop big numbers one week yet stay the same or even go up a pound the next. Don't let that derail you. Consistent effort over time is what ensures a lifetime of good health.

Weight loss is a process. It's never a straight path to your goal. Some weeks you may drop big numbers, and other weeks you may plateau or even gain a pound or two. This is perfectly normal. Weight loss is always faster in the beginning, because that's when you have more to lose, but it slows down as you get closer to your goal. We see jaw-dropping numbers the first week the contestants step on the scale at the Ranch because they are being medically supervised, are on a calorie regimen, and go from zero to 60 mph in terms of activity, and thus lose a ton of water weight. You should not strive for such rapid results at home—unless you have on-site, 24-hour-a-day medical experts, as the *Biggest Losers* do!

As you lose weight, your calorie requirement is going to drop—a bit. Don't panic. We're talking about tweaking your calorie intake as needed, not slashing and burning.

It takes a lot of calories to fuel fat. For every pound of fat you lose, you decrease the number of calories you expend each day by about 10. That's roughly the number of calories that were required to keep that fat at body temperature, move it around, and support its metabolic needs. So when you shed 10 pounds of fat, you will be burning about 100 calories fewer each day than you did when you weighed more. If you want to keep losing weight, you have to make some adjustments.

Contestants even have to pay attention to what they eat in *The Biggest Loser* kitchen. "Watch out for the peanut butter!" Season 5 winner Ali Vincent always warns new contestants. "A spoonful here, a spoonful there—if you're not writing it down, it can bite you. I got almost superstitious during my season. I'd see someone in the kitchen dipping that spoon in the peanut butter jar once, twice . . . and then they'd get eliminated!"

At the Ranch, all the contestants have homework. They tally up their daily calorie intakes. If they don't have the right balance of calories in/calories out, they will burn what they need to by getting in an extra workout, taking a walk, or hopping in the pool for a quick lap or two.

When to Eat

On *The Biggest Loser* plan, you'll eat five or six meals each day, including three main meals (breakfast, lunch, and dinner) and two or three snacks. Parceling out your calories through the day means you'll stay full and won't go on sugar or carb binges to satisfy your growling stomach. It also means you won't go to bed feeling stuffed and sick from too many bad, empty calories. Ed Brantley of Season 6, a professional chef, used to eat his first meal of the day at lunchtime, when he'd scarf down a few burgers. It started a cycle of bad choices that lasted throughout the day.

Eating more-frequent meals and snacks will:

- Keep you from feeling deprived.
- Help control blood sugar and insulin levels (insulin is a fat-forming hormone).
- Lead to lower body fat.
- Keep you energized for exercise and activity.
- Reduce stress hormones in the body that can contribute to fat accumulation.
- Establish a regular pattern of eating that helps counter impulse eating.

"At first, I really had to work to get all my meals in," recalls Danny Cahill, the Season 8 winner. "I wasn't used to eating healthy. I quickly realized that nutrient-dense foods were more satisfying than all the fat I was getting from fast food. It kept up my energy level, and I felt fueled for workouts."

Even if you work at night, which plenty of contestants do, it's important to eat a small meal within 30 minutes of waking, especially if you're going to get your workout in before you go to work. And then go from there. Just shift your meals accordingly.

You Skip, You Gain

Contestants arriving at the Ranch are often surprised to learn that one reason they've gained so much weight is that they've had a habit of skipping meals, just like Ed Brantley. Skipping meals can actually contribute to weight *gain,* not loss.

One recent study conducted by the National Institute on Aging indicated that people who skipped meals during the day and ate all their calories at one nightly meal showed unhealthy changes in their metabolism, similar to unhealthy blood sugar levels observed in people with diabetes.

Non–meal skippers, on the other hand, consumed the same number of calories, but distributed them throughout the day at three regular meal intervals. The people who ate regular meals maintained healthy blood sugar levels. But healthy blood sugar levels aren't the only reason to plan regular meals and snacks.

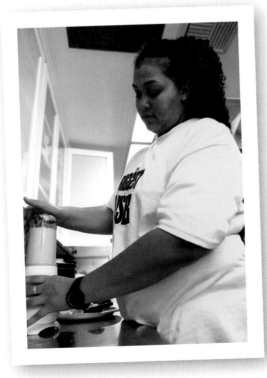

Get a Clue about Hunger Cues

Another problem with skipping meals is that by the time mealtime rolls around, you're famished. Just like Ed and his burgers-for-breakfast routine, contestants who don't eat all day make the worst choices. Fat has more than twice as many calories as protein and carbohydrate. It satisfies hunger very quickly, and your body seems to know this. So the longer you go without food, the more likely you are to crave a fat-filled treat.

The other problem with skipping meals is that when you wait too long to eat, you lose sight of your body's natural hunger cues. You don't really know when you're hungry anymore (or when you're full). Most overeaters don't stop eating when they're comfortable—they stop when they're stuffed!

From starving to stuffed, the hunger scale on the opposite page defines your body's hunger signals and how to interpret them.

The Biggest Loser Hunger Scale

1. **Famished or starving:** You feel weak and/or lightheaded. This is a big no-no.

2. **Very hungry:** You can't think of anything else but eating. You're cranky and irritable and can't concentrate.

3. **Hungry:** Your stomach's growling and feels empty.

4. **A little bit hungry:** You're just starting to think about your next meal.

5. **Satisfied:** You're comfortable, not really thinking about food. You feel alert and have a good energy level.

6. **Fully satisfied:** You've had enough to eat, maybe a little too much. Maybe you took a few extra bites for taste only, not hunger.

7. **Very full:** Now you need to unzip your jeans. You're uncomfortable, bloated, tired. Maybe you don't feel great. Where's the couch . . . ? You should never feel like this after a meal.

Hunger Scale Flash Card

1–3: Eat! Eat!

5: Stop, especially if you're trying to lose weight.

6: Definitely stop.

7: You may have waited too long. Better go find the couch and start over tomorrow.

Weighing and Measuring

We all know that serving sizes can be tricky, especially when it comes to processed foods. No, a bag of popcorn is not one serving. *Warning:* If a processed food comes in one package, chances are that one package holds multiple servings. The number of servings is listed in the tiny print on the back label. Learn to read the label.

Even when you are cooking healthy food in your kitchen—such as the recipes in this book—you need to know how much food qualifies as a serving in order to accurately track your calories. To do so, you will need to equip your kitchen with:

- Liquid measuring cup (2-cup capacity)
- Set of dry measuring cups (includes 1-cup, ½-cup, ⅓-cup, and ¼-cup sizes)
- Measuring spoons (1 tablespoon, 1 teaspoon, ½ teaspoon, and ¼ teaspoon)
- *The Biggest Loser* Food Scale
- Calculator

Conversion Table for Measuring Portion Sizes

Teaspoons	Tablespoons	Cups	Pints, quarts, gallons	Fluid ounces	Milliliters
¼ teaspoon					1 ml
½ teaspoon					2 ml
1 teaspoon	⅓ tablespoon				5 ml
3 teaspoons	1 tablespoon	⅟₁₆ cup		½ oz	15 ml
6 teaspoons	2 tablespoons	⅛ cup		1 oz	30 ml
12 teaspoons	4 tablespoons	¼ cup		2 oz	60 ml
16 teaspoons	5⅓ tablespoons	⅓ cup		2½ oz	75 ml
24 teaspoons	8 tablespoons	½ cup		4 oz	125 ml
32 teaspoons	10⅔ tablespoons	⅔ cup		5 oz	150 ml
36 teaspoons	12 tablespoons	¾ cup		6 oz	175 ml
48 teaspoons	16 tablespoons	1 cup	½ pint	8 oz	237 ml
		2 cups	1 pint	16 oz	473 ml
		3 cups		24 oz	710 ml
		4 cups	1 quart	32 oz	946 ml
		8 cups	½ gallon	64 oz	
		16 cups	1 gallon	128 oz	

Be sure that the food scale measures grams. (A gram is very small, about ¹⁄₂₈ of an ounce.) Most of your weight measurements will be in ounces, but certain foods, such as nuts, are very concentrated in calories, so you may need to measure your portion size in grams. You can also rely on *The Biggest Loser Calorie Counter* to calculate calories when you're at work or on the go.

Most *Biggest Loser* contestants learn some visual cues for measuring or eyeballing portion sizes. And you can do the same thing—the only "tool" you need is your hand!

- Fist = 1 cup of fruit or 1 medium whole, raw fruit
- Thumb = 1 ounce of cheese or meat
- Fingertip = approximately 1 teaspoon
- Tip of thumb = approximately 1 tablespoon
- One cupped hand = 1 or 2 ounces of dry goods (nuts, cereal, pretzels)

For consistency, weigh or measure your food *after* cooking. Four ounces of boneless, skinless chicken breast has around 140 calories when raw. When it's cooked, it will weigh closer to 3 ounces. That's because it loses water during the cooking process, and the calories are now more concentrated. The same holds true for vegetables and other cooked foods. Dry cereals or grains, on the other hand, may start off at a couple of tablespoons per serving. When you add water and cook them, the volume or measured amount may double or triple.

After measuring all your foods for a week or so, you'll be able to make fairly accurate estimates by eye without having to measure everything each time you eat. Of course, you'll always need to weigh and measure when trying a food for the first time, so keep your measuring tools in a handy location. Over time, you'll know what's just right for you, whether you're plating a meal in your own kitchen or deciding how much of your entrée to eat in a restaurant (and how much of it to wrap up and take home!). But in the beginning, you'll need a few tools until you get it just right.

If you're not accustomed to spending time in the kitchen, the conversion table on the opposite page may be helpful to you.

Remember that an ounce of weight is not the same as a fluid ounce. You cannot convert the two without knowing the density of the ingredient you are measuring.

Write It All Down!

Though the contestants at the Ranch *have* to keep a food journal, this is one practice that most *Biggest Losers* maintain for life. At the Season 8 finale, all of the contestants were asked how they planned to continue and maintain their weight loss. Every single one of them mentioned food journaling as an essential part of their strategy.

Once your daily calorie budget is established, record your food and beverage intake daily. Faithfully keeping a calorie budget and a food journal will direct you toward discovering the most favorable foods for your eating strategy—those that leave you satisfied. Exploring new food and recipe possibilities is one key to mastering this approach. Another key tactic is recognizing and avoiding appetite-stimulating foods (usually processed foods with high starch, sugar, and/or fat content) and trigger foods that lead to excessively large portions.

As you learn which foods work best for you, make sure those foods are around when you need them. Eat those foods at home and, whenever possible, bring them with you when you go to work or travel. Similarly, try to keep trigger foods out of your home environment.

Keeping a food journal is paramount to your successful weight-loss plan. It will help you identify the times that you eat certain things, allowing you to learn from your eating patterns. It is imperative to keep track of the number of calories you take in and burn off through exercise each day, especially when you're just getting started. Buy a notebook and a pen just for this purpose, and keep them in your desk, your handbag, or your backpack, or record this information on your computer—whatever is handy or convenient. Take notes throughout the day, otherwise it's easy to forget an unplanned snack or tasting. Create a routine: Find a favorite place and time to record in your journal.

You can reference the sample format on the opposite page to create your own food journal.

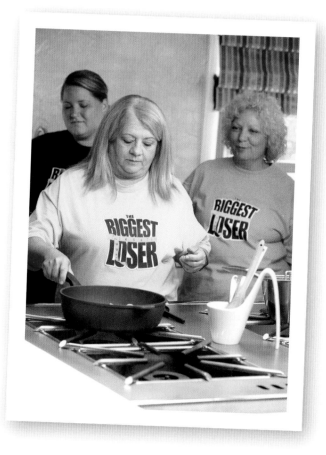

Sample Food Journal Page

	Calories	Carbohydrate (45%)	Protein (30%)	Fat (25%)
Sample Goal	1,200	540	360	300

Meal/ Time	Food	Calories	Carbohydrate	Protein	Fat
	Totals				
	Goal Totals				
	+/-				

Quality Calories

Like most overweight Americans, many of *The Biggest Loser* contestants come to the Ranch with a history of eating and drinking too much of the wrong types of foods and beverages and eating too little of the right kinds of foods. In a nutshell, they don't pay enough attention to what or how much they eat at any given time, from snacks to meals.

It's not uncommon to meet contestants who eat all three meals out, often at fast-food outlets. The bad thing about convenience eating is that when you're not making your food, you can't control how it's prepared. Sione Fa confessed in Season 7 that he would pick up fast-food tacos on the way home—before sitting down to dinner! (His wife didn't find out until later.) And Mike Morelli, also of Season 7, was so embarrassed about his fast-food fix that he would swing by the fast-food place, pick up a couple of cheeseburgers, and scarf down the evidence before getting home—all in a span of 10 minutes.

Most of these excess calories are empty calories—that is, they lack nutrient value and don't contain vitamins, minerals, or the powerful antioxidants that help ward off disease. The American diet is full of the wrong kinds of foods, and eating too many of these foods can increase your chances of getting sick—from catching the common cold to developing high blood pressure. Eating too much of the wrong stuff will also leave you with less energy, mentally and physically. Many *Biggest Losers* come to the Ranch with complaints of being tired all the time. The reason? Poor diet and not enough exercise!

Even after just a few days on the Ranch, contestants start feeling better from "clean eating." They find that they no longer press the snooze button in

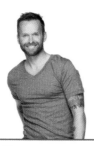

Biggest Loser Trainer Tip: Bob Harper

You can go out to dinner and still eat healthfully. Just remember to plan ahead. Visit the restaurant's online menu and decide ahead of time what you want to order so that you bypass those last-minute temptations. Avoid anything on the menu that is sautéed or pan-fried. Instead, order your food grilled, steamed, baked, broiled, or poached.

the morning—they wake up feeling full of energy. The Season 9 contestants described the change in their energy levels as "night and day."

Here are some of the main culprits in the average *Biggest Loser's* pre-Ranch diet.

- Red meat, fast foods, and processed foods are consumed at all hours.
- Loads of cholesterol, salt, and sugar are added to the mix.
- Not enough fresh fruits and vegetables are consumed.
- Fiber and antioxidants are at a bare minimum.
- Drink of choice is soda, soda, and more soda.
- Chaotic schedules result in many skipped meals and/or eating on the run.

At the Ranch, the contestants learn to:

- Veggie-load in every way possible, with salads, sandwiches, and sides.
- Amp up their fruit intake by skipping sugary juices and adding fresh fruit to smoothies.
- Love and learn to pronounce quinoa (KEEN-wah)—it's a grain *and* a protein!
- Eat lean cuts of meat and poultry and increase fish intake to several times a week. Salmon and orange roughy are Ranch favorites.

- Eat open-faced sandwiches with one slice of Ezekiel bread, full of fiber.
- Select whole grains such as brown rice and whole wheat pasta.
- Minimize consumption of red meat and high-fat dairy foods.

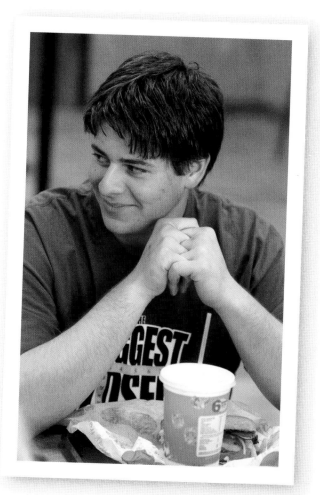

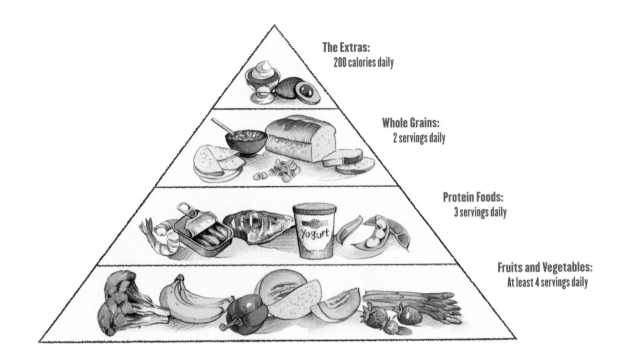

The Extras:
200 calories daily

Whole Grains:
2 servings daily

Protein Foods:
3 servings daily

Fruits and Vegetables:
At least 4 servings daily

The Biggest Loser Plan: Building the Pyramid

45 Percent of Your Daily Calories

Complex Carbohydrates— Vegetables, Fruits, Whole Grains

Aim for a minimum of 4 cups of a variety of fruits and nonstarchy vegetables daily. Favor fruits (fresh, not dried) and nonstarchy vegetables over grain products. Choose whole grain foods in moderation, and select those with high fiber content.

Vegetables

- Cook your vegetables for the least amount of time possible to preserve nutrients.
- Avoid added fat; steam, grill, or stir-fry veggies in a nonstick pan.
- Try to eat at least one vegetable raw each day.
- Eat a vegetable salad most days of the week.
- Plan ahead—keep cut-up vegetables such as bell

peppers, broccoli, and jicama in your fridge for easy snacking at home or to take to work or school.

- Starchier vegetables such as pumpkin, winter squash, and sweet potatoes are higher in calories and carbs, so limit them to a serving or two per week.

- Fresh vegetables are best, but it's perfectly okay to choose frozen. If you opt for canned, watch the sodium content. You need to rinse canned vegetables before eating to wash away added salt.

Fruits

- Enjoy at least one raw fruit each day. Try a new fruit every week to add variety to your diet.

- Dark green, light green, orange, purple, red, and yellow: Savor fruits from different color groups. This ensures you're getting a variety of nutrients.

- Eat fruit for dessert! Many *Biggest Losers* who have a sweet tooth use this strategy. Try indulging in sweet, tropical fruits like kiwi and mango instead of eating a slice of cake or a bowl of ice cream.

- Dried fruits are more concentrated in calories and sugar than raw fruits, and they're not as filling. Cup for cup, fresh grapes have only a fourth of the calories found in raisins. Opt for fresh fruit whenever possible, though you

can add flavor—and a serving of fruit—by adding chopped dried fruit to grain dishes like couscous and quinoa, to vegetable salads, and to meat dishes like **Moroccan Pork Stew with Baby Artichokes and Dried Fruit** (page 112).

- Choose whole fruit rather than fruit juices. Fruit juice contains less fiber, so it's not as filling as whole fruit, and it's more concentrated in sugars, so it will cause a spike in your blood sugar. When you do choose juice, remember that a serving size is 4 ounces (½ cup).

- Fresh fruit is preferable, but frozen fruit is fine as long as it's not packaged with added sugar or syrup. If you choose canned fruit, be sure it's packed in water.

Whole Grains

Whole grains are those that have undergone minimal processing and thus have retained most of their nutritional value. When whole grains are refined, important nutrients are removed. All that's usually left is starch, which is loaded with carbohydrate calories and little else. Whole grains can sometimes be found in bulk bins at your grocery store. Since you're not paying for expensive packaging and labels, significant cost savings—up to 50 percent or more—can be passed on to you.

When choosing bread products, read the label

carefully. If it says "enriched," the product probably contains white flour—meaning it's low in fiber and nutrition. Choose breads with at least 2 grams of fiber per serving, but aim for 5 grams. In the ingredient list, the first item should be "whole wheat" or "whole grain." "Wheat flour" isn't necessarily whole wheat; the term usually means enriched flour with some whole wheat added.

Most packaged breakfast cereals are highly processed and loaded with added sugar. Choose packaged cereals with fewer than 5 grams of sugar and at least 5 grams of fiber per serving.

Protein

Remember to include protein with each meal and snack so your body can use it throughout the day. There's plenty to choose from in three different protein groups: animal protein, low-fat (or fat-free) dairy protein, and vegetarian protein. Often, when contestants start to feel hungry, nutritionist Cheryl Forberg realizes they're not pairing protein with fruit, for example, for a snack.

- Choose a variety of proteins each day to meet your calorie goal.

Eat Out with Whole Grains!

Here are some tips for making whole grain choices at a restaurant.

- If you haven't eliminated bread from your diet, ask for whole grain rolls, crackers, or tortillas (corn or whole wheat) instead of white.

- Choose old-fashioned or steel-cut oatmeal or whole grain bagels for breakfast.

- Ask for brown rice instead of white rice.

- Ask to substitute whole wheat pasta in a pasta dish.

- Choose whole grain dishes such as polenta, brown rice, wild rice, bulgur, and tabbouleh for your starch instead of potatoes or white rice.

- If your favorite restaurant doesn't offer any whole grain choices, keep asking! If enough customers are interested, you may be in for a pleasant surprise the next time you go back. Restaurants want to keep their customers happy and returning, so make your desires known. Unless we request more nutritious carbohydrates when we dine out, refined products (white stuff) will probably remain the standard.

- Limit your servings of lean red meat to twice a week. Red meat tends to be higher in saturated fat.
- Fish is an excellent source of protein, omega-3 fatty acids, vitamin E, and selenium. Cold-water fish contain more heart-healthy fats—they also have more calories.
- Avoid processed meats, such as bologna, hot dogs, and sausage. They're generally high in fat and calories, and they may also contain sodium nitrites, which can form carcinogenic (potentially cancer-causing) compounds (see Chapter 6 for more information).

Animal Protein

Meat

Choose lean cuts of meat, such as pork tenderloin and beef round, chuck, sirloin, or tenderloin. USDA Choice or USDA Select grades of beef usually have lower fat content. Avoid meat that is heavily marbled and remove any visible fat. Try to find ground meat that is at least 95 percent lean.

Poultry

The leanest poultry is the skinless white meat from the breast of chicken or turkey. When purchasing ground chicken or turkey, ask for the white meat.

Seafood

Select fish and seafood (especially wild varieties) that are rich in omega-3 fatty acids. This includes salmon, sardines (water packed), herring, mackerel, trout, and tuna.

Dairy

Top choices include fat-free (skim) milk, 1% (low-fat) milk, buttermilk, plain fat-free or low-fat yogurt, fat-free or low-fat yogurt with fruit (no sugar added), fat-free or low-fat cottage cheese, and fat-free or low-fat ricotta cheese. Light soy milks and soy yogurts can also be used, but if you eat soy because of a dairy intolerance or allergy, be sure to select soy products that are fortified with calcium. Egg whites are also an excellent fat-free source of protein. And if you're not getting three servings of dairy per day, *The Biggest Loser* nutrition team recommends taking a calcium supplement.

Vegetarian Protein

Excellent sources of vegetarian protein include beans, other legumes, and traditional soy foods, such as tofu and edamame. Many of these foods are loaded with fiber.

25 Percent of Your Daily Calories

Good Fats

This is not a license to eat any form of fat you want. Many of the fat calories you derive from healthy fats will be hidden in your carbohydrate and protein food choices. You will have a small budget of leftover calories to spend on healthy fat and "extras." Healthy fats include small servings of nuts and seeds and an occasional spray or splash of olive oil or canola oil for your salads or cooked dishes.

Many of *The Biggest Losers* like to allocate a small number of calories (100 to 150) for extras. Try to spend these on healthy food choices instead of candy or sweets. Your meals should be made up mostly of whole foods, with less emphasis on "diet food" substitutes. Healthy choices include a few healthy fats each day, such as nuts and seeds, sugar-free (or reduced-sugar) sweets or desserts,

A Healthy Dinner to Go

During Season 8, the kitchen was locked down for 1 week, and the contestants had to order out for every meal—breakfast, lunch, and dinner. How did they cope? Here are some tips they sent to BiggestLoserClub.com about how they stayed on track.

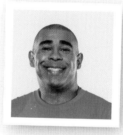

Try ordering à la carte to avoid this situation. Pick out main components— a side of steamed veggies or brown rice.

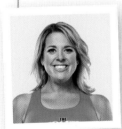

Abby Rike

Decide what you're in the mood for. Then make modifications to the menu that's available to you. Be specific about how you want your food prepared. It can make a big difference.

Allen Smith

If you order out and they bring the food to you and it's not what you ordered, you can't fix it.

Amanda Arlauskas

Having someone else prepare food for you can be tough. Ask about every ingredient that's in the dish that you want. Or just ask for exactly what you want. If you want grilled chicken and steamed veggies, ask for that. And ask what they cook with—grease, oil, lard? Extra calories can sneak in, and you won't even realize it.

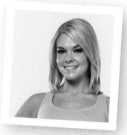

and low-sugar and low-sodium condiments. Take advantage of herbs and spices to add flavor to your foods.

To get the biggest bang out of your calorie budget, limit your extras and stick to the whole foods in this plan. You'll be happy you did when you step on the scale!

Decoding Food Labels

Just because a product looks healthy doesn't mean it is. Pay special attention to the calories on "light," "reduced-fat," "low-fat," and "fat-free" products. When the fat is removed from many recipes, salt and sugar are added to boost flavor. This can

Daniel Wright
When ordering restaurant food, get creative. Order corn instead of flour tortillas. Look at the menu and see what you can do to lighten up the options.

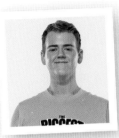

Danny Cahill
You have to specify exactly how you want your food cooked. You have to choose what to do. When I order an omelet, I tell them I don't want any butter or oil.

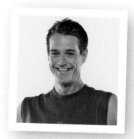

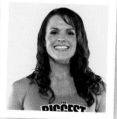

Dina Mercado
When you buy takeout, make sure you check your food before you leave the restaurant, because you don't always get what you order. If

you get home and you notice something wasn't cooked the way you wanted it, just portion it out. Be wise about how much of it you eat.

Liz Young
If you're not able to eat healthy all the time, just be aware of the calories you're taking in. But you can't eat unhealthy food every day and expect to lose weight. You have to exercise to burn off the extra calories.

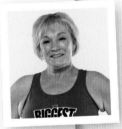

Tracey Yukich
Make sure you are precise with your ordering technique. If you want salad, specify romaine lettuce or spring mix. Keep one-half of your plate full of veggies, one-quarter protein, one-quarter complex carbs.

result in a fat-free or low-fat product that actually has *more* calories (and/or sugar and/or salt) than the regular version.

Here's a quick guide to decoding packaging promises:

- *Organic* foods have been grown without the use of pesticides, which means they can be much better for you, especially when it comes to whole fruits and vegetables. But be careful with packaged foods: Just because the ingredients are organic does not necessarily mean the product is healthy. Some candy is organic!
- *Reduced calorie* means the food contains at least 25 percent fewer calories than the regular version—but it doesn't guarantee it will be good for *your* calorie budget!
- *Low calorie* means the product contains no more than 40 calories per serving (except sugar substitutes).
- *Reduced fat* means that a product has 25 percent less fat than the regular counterpart—but that could still be quite a bit of fat.
- *Light* means a product has 50 percent less fat than its regular counterpart. Again, it's better than nothing, but double-check the grams of fat per serving to see what that 50 percent adds up to.
- *Low fat* means there are 3 grams of fat (or less) in a serving. Products with this label are usually a good bet.
- *Fat free* means the product contains a half gram of fat (or less) per serving. Just double-check the calories to make sure they didn't pile on the sugar.
- *Light in sodium* means this product has half the sodium of its traditional counterpart. Again, that is a good sign, but check for actual milligrams per serving—the product may still be high in sodium.

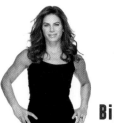

Biggest Loser Trainer Tip: Jillian Michaels

Sandwiches make for a healthy meal, but not when they're loaded with mayonnaise and cheese. The next time you make a sandwich, skip the unhealthy condiments and instead use avocado. Spreading ¼ cup of avocado on your bread will make your sandwich taste great—plus the avocado has healthier fat and fewer calories.

Superfoods: Top 10 Foods for Health

Not all the vitamins and nutrients you need for optimum health are stored by the body. Our bodies can store fat-soluble vitamins such as A, D, and E as well as essential omega fatty acids, but water-soluble vitamins such as B (including thiamin, riboflavin, niacin, and folate) and C stay in the bloodstream for only 4 to 6 hours. To maintain optimal blood levels of important nutrients, you should eat a variety of the following superfoods *throughout the day,* not just at one meal. And remember—supplements are supplemental. Real food is the winning ticket for a strong and healthy body!

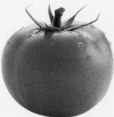

1. Tomatoes

Tomatoes contain tons of vitamins A and C and something called lycopene, a plant chemical that helps protect our bodies against cancer and our skin against UV damage from the sun. Lycopene is concentrated when tomatoes are cooked. Cooking tomatoes with a small amount of oil increases lycopene absorption by the body.

2. Bell peppers

Low in calories and loaded with antioxidants; one whole bell pepper has only 30 calories and twice your daily requirement of vitamin C.

3. Avocado

Good fats like those found in avocados help your body absorb fat-soluble vitamins. The avocado's beautiful green color indicates the presence of the plant chemical lutein, which is stored in the maculae of our eyes and promotes eye health. A 1-ounce serving of avocado has 50 calories— less than in a tablespoon of mayonnaise.

4. Beans and other legumes

The powerhouse legume family includes hundreds of beans, peas, peanuts, and lentils that are all excellent sources of fiber. They're also rich in folic acid, calcium, iron, potassium, zinc, and antioxidants. Their high protein and complex carbohydrate profiles provide steady energy that lasts for hours. And a daily serving of cooked beans may lower blood cholesterol by as much as 18 percent!

Beans also contain prebiotics, nutrients that are used by specific strains of bacteria. When added to the diet, prebiotics increase the chances of beneficial bacteria growth in the intestine.

Many beans, especially white ones, contain resistant starch. Like prebiotics, this starch is attacked by good bacteria and fermented in a process thought to initiate anticancer benefits. Lentils are the most underrated legume—loaded with vitamins, nutrients, protein, and fiber, they take only 20 minutes to cook and are an inexpensive form of protein. A half cup of cooked lentils contains 9 grams of protein and 8 grams of fiber.

5. Wild salmon and other cold-water fish

Salmon contains omega-3 fatty acids, which are essential fats not produced by our bodies. Omega-3s are vital for brain function, healthy skin and hair, and well-tuned cardiovascular and nervous systems. Omega-3s are also found in seaweed, watercress, flaxseed, walnuts, and almonds. The plant forms take longer to convert to the active form of fat our bodies need, so cold-water fish (such as wild salmon, mackerel, and herring) are the best sources of omega-3s.

6. Lean proteins

Though they don't have the antioxidants and vitamins of plant foods, lean proteins contain micronutrients (such as calcium, iron, selenium, and zinc) that are essential not only for bone formation and nerve transmission but for fighting cancer,

forming blood cells, and keeping our immune systems robust.

Lean proteins repair tissue, build and preserve muscle, and make important enzymes and hormones.

7. Whole grains

The grain family includes barley, corn, millet, oats, brown rice, rye, and wheat. Amaranth, buckwheat, and quinoa are also called whole grains, although technically they are seeds. Whole grains offer protein, B vitamins, minerals, dietary fiber, and antioxidants (such as lignans and phenolic acids) that help protect against heart disease, some cancers, obesity, and diabetes. Old-fashioned or steel-cut oatmeal (not the instant or quick-cooking varieties) contains plenty of beta-glucan fiber, which binds to cholesterol in the intestinal tract, thus contributing to lowered LDL (bad cholesterol). It also moderates the release of glucose into the bloodstream, improving blood sugar control.

8. Greek-style yogurt

This delicious, creamy treat is a favorite at the Ranch. Greek-style yogurt is strained more than typical American-style yogurts, which removes more of the yogurt's watery whey. Since whey is mostly carbohydrate (with a small amount of protein), the strained yogurt contains less carbohydrate and more protein. One cup of plain, fat-free Greek-style yogurt has approximately 100 calories, 5 grams of carbohydrate, and 20 grams of protein. In comparison, 1 cup of plain, fat-free American-style yogurt contains approximately 100 calories, 19 grams of carbohydrate, and 10 grams of protein. The tanginess of Greek-style yogurt makes it a perfect substitute for sour cream in savory dips and spreads.

9. Berries

All whole fruits are excellent sources of nutrients, but berries stand out from the pack. Fresh berries can give your memory a boost as well as protect your body against cancer and heart disease. Berries contain antioxidants such as anthocyanin, which has triple the power of vitamin C and is known to block cancer-causing damage and the effects of many age-related diseases. Fresh berries are better than dried if you're watching your weight, because the fresh berries' water content makes them more filling, and the vitamins are at their peak when the berries are freshly picked.

Strawberries rank with oranges in terms of vitamin C content and are a real immunity booster. Other great choices are raspberries, blueberries, and blackberries.

10. Nuts and seeds

It's true that most of the calories in nuts come from fat, but our bodies need some of these fats. In conjunction with a diet of fresh fruits and vegetables, lean protein, and whole grains, nuts provide protection from heart disease and help reduce blood pressure. Many nuts contain phytosterols, the "cholesterol clones" that promote heart health and may prevent colon cancer. All varieties of nuts—such as almonds, walnuts, pistachios, pecans, hazelnuts, and Brazil nuts—are also rich in protein.

Seeds are another calorie-dense but healthy source of protein and other nutrients, when eaten in moderation. Sesame seeds, especially, are an excellent source of calcium and heart-healthy fats. They contain several forms of vitamin E, which are believed to play a role in the prevention of aging-related diseases such as heart disease and cancer.

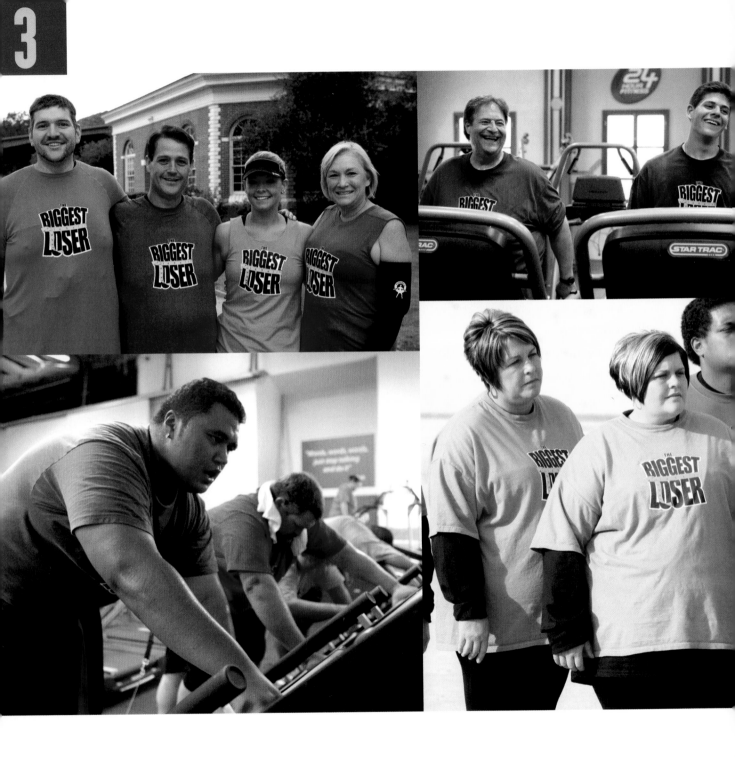

3

Reclaim Your Life

You watch *The Biggest Losers* undergo dramatic transformations at the Ranch—but do you ever wonder how their experiences on campus impact their lives at home? We caught up with past contestants to find out how losing weight has changed their lives. One of the questions we asked each of them was "After losing so much weight—what have you gained?" The response we received was universal: "Life."

The Season 8 contestants are already seeing their hard work pay off in the form of major life changes. Winner Danny Cahill certainly got his life back as he reclaimed his former rockin' self, the fit and handsome musician who used to have the world at his feet. Now he can be the father and husband he always wanted to be for his family. Now he can play with his kids and set an example for a young daughter who, until recently, wanted to be just like her dad, big belly and all.

After losing weight and regaining her confidence,

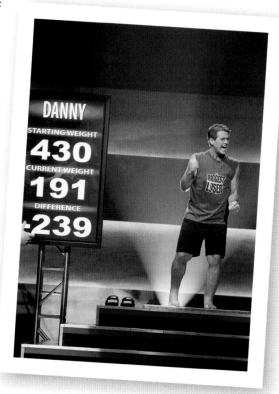

Season 8 finalist Amanda Arlauskas says she's ready to start dating and find the love of her life. The 20-year-old admits that her weight kept her from attending her high school prom. Now Allen Smith doesn't have to make excuses to get out of running around with his daughter in the front yard—and as a fireman, he doesn't have to worry that he won't be able to help someone who desperately needs to be rescued. And the newly engaged Antoine Dove and Alexandra White can start building a healthy, active future together and enjoy each other's companionship for many years to come.

Season 7's Cathy Skell says she's gotten her life back in every way imaginable now that she's healthy. "I am happier. I no longer look in the mirror in disgust; I was my own worst critic. I have 20 years of sobriety along with my weight loss. What a wonderful combination! I now have my self-esteem back.

"I battled alcohol at age 29 and my weight loss at age 49," continues Cathy. "The sad thing is that at age 49, weighing in at 293 pounds, I was a mother and a grandmother of three, and I accepted my weight for what it was. I could only *think* what I wanted; I never actually *tried*, because I assumed that with high blood pressure and asthma, I could never run, jog, or exercise to break a sweat. I am so proud of my accomplishments and love to share with anyone who is strug-

gling that you *can* change your life, no matter what age you are!"

Now, Cathy says, she's made a resolution to change her life and be healthier. "In regards to every decision that I've made, is this ultimately going to lead me to my goal of health. When it came to temptations, I had to keep my eye on the prize. Health is my prize; that's where my eye is.

"Every decision you are faced with is a choice," she concludes. "It's just a matter of making the right choices."

First Stop: Dr. Huizenga

If you've watched *The Biggest Loser,* you've probably seen Dr. Robert Huizenga (frequently referred to by the contestants as Dr. H), the resident medical expert on *The Biggest Loser* campus. He's the guy who delivers tough news to contestants about the true state of their health, something many of them have been in denial about until they hear him state the cold, hard facts.

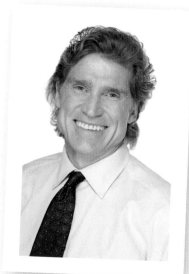

"No one had ever taken sedentary couch potatoes and conditioned them like you condition pro athletes," says Dr. Huizenga. "Season 1, we were very, very nervous. I lost a lot of sleep." Now, he says, he has become used to the fact that most of the contestants arrive at the Ranch unaware that "they are at high risk for a litany of diseases."

Dr. Huizenga and his team have "made it okay to be fat and to work out." Excuses stop at Dr. Huizenga's office. Season 5 winner Ali Vincent says she thought she would never have to run at the Ranch—something she used to hate—because she'd had knee surgeries. "I thought it was my 'get out of jail free' card," she laughed, "but Dr. Huiz-

Scary Health Care Stats

Did you know that health care is the largest industry in the United States, with over *$2 trillion* spent on medical care? That dollar amount is approaching 16 percent of the nation's gross domestic product (GDP)—and it's expected to reach over $4 trillion by 2015. That would be 20 percent of our GDP!

According to the Centers for Disease Control and Prevention (CDC), 70 percent of the money we spend on health care in America is associated with preventable conditions such as chronic heart disease, stroke, and type 2 diabetes. The common denominator among all these diseases? Obesity.

Two-thirds of Americans are considered obese, and 80 percent of the country's total health care expenditures are tied to only 20 percent of the people. For example,

18.2 million Americans have diabetes. It's estimated there are another 5.5 million who are undiagnosed. And more than 40 million Americans are prediabetic and at high risk for developing the disease. Once diagnosed, treatment for diabetes costs an estimated $10,000 per patient per year.

Ask yourself these questions to start getting a better picture of your health:

1. Are you more than 10 pounds overweight?
2. Do you frequently miss your annual checkup?
3. Do you exercise less than 30 minutes per day, four or five times per week?
4. Are you unaware of your blood pressure and cholesterol numbers?
5. Are you interested in a healthier lifestyle but looking for a place to start?

enga looked at my medical history and said that wasn't true. I could run. And I did. Now I run all the time!"

One of Dr. Huizenga's biggest surprises was Season 6's Jerry Skeabeck. "I wasn't sure he was going to make it alive to the end of the show, much less make a successful transformation," he remembers. When Dr. H sat Jerry down early in the season, he put it to him straight. He said, "You've got every risk factor known to medicine." At 51, Jerry was told his body's real age was 76. It took a few weeks for Jerry to be able to fully participate in exercise, but once he did, Dr. Huizenga notes, "he caught fire."

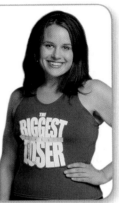

Jerry started his season at 380 pounds. After losing more than 100 pounds, Jerry is living more comfortably at 262. "We all get rude awakenings in our life," says Jerry. "Some come sooner, and some come later. I felt that mine came later. At 51 years old, the day that Dr. H told me how old I was internally, it hit me when I saw my daughter [teammate Coleen] cry.

I realized I have a family that means a lot to me and me to them. I thought, 'What does it take for me to wake up?'"

Dr. Huizenga says that for most *Biggest Loser* contestants who come to the Ranch with preexisting health conditions, exercise-focused weight loss has been a "magic bullet." He adds, "The thoroughness and eradication of symptoms . . . I've got to admit, as a doctor, it's been a bit of a shocker for me."

When Jerry arrived at the Ranch, he was taking medicine for high blood pressure and for his heart arrhythmia. After just 6 weeks of exercise and healthy eating, he no longer needed any medication, and he is pill free to this day.

Each season the contestants undergo a battery of medical exams so that Dr. H can get an accurate picture of their health and their potential for developing disease. The Season 9 contestants were the first ever to use the Know Your Number Health-Score tool, which provided them with detailed information about their Inner Age—or the rate at which their bodies were aging due to unhealthy lifestyles—as well as their risk of developing of major chronic diseases. And more important, the Know Your Number tool also showed them the best ways to reduce their risk and get healthy.

Inspiring Others

Biggest Loser contestants don't just change their own lives—they inspire others to get healthy, too. Season 2 contestant Pete Thomas has made this his lifelong mission. Weighing in at 401 pounds when he arrived on campus, today he weighs a healthy

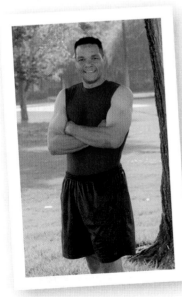

238. "I'm often asked how my life is different after versus before *The Biggest Loser.* I like to say that I simply look on the outside like I've always felt on the inside. I believe that I've been given a unique gift—my health, my life back. So I'm paying it forward to

enable other people to have a new lease on life. I've developed a 10-week series of classes called Lose It Fast, Lose It Forever. I love to see people work out incredibly hard and do more than they think they can do. There's a certain amount of pride in being able to share this with others."

Drea Baptiste of Season 1 has used her *Biggest Loser* experience to build a new career. Stepping on *The Biggest Loser* scale at 215 pounds when she first arrived at the Ranch, today she weighs 160. "Since losing the weight, my life has been absolutely phenomenal. I am able to do so much more and empowered to do so

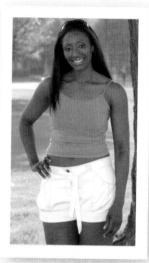

much more," she says. Drea is now the director of a nonprofit organization that works with inner-city women and children who wouldn't necessarily be able to afford gym memberships.

"It has been such a tremendous journey to go through my challenges and to conquer them," says Drea. "I can do anything I set my heart on, and I can get it done. I'm going to keep going on and on until I feel I've conquered all there is for me to conquer."

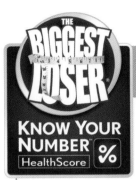

Health Score Quiz

Below is a self-assessment quiz you can take at home to determine your risk factors for developing disease. It's a good idea to take the quiz now and then retake it after you've completed the 6-week program, so that you can track your progress.

Questions

1. What is your gender?
   a. Female
   b. Male

2. How old are you?
   a. Younger than 50
   b. 50 or older

3. What is your ethnicity?
   a. White
   b. Black or Latino
   c. Asian
   d. None of the above

4. How many times a week do you exercise for at least 20 minutes at a time?
   a. 5 or more
   b. 2 to 4
   c. 1 or fewer

5. While exercising, how hard are you breathing?
   a. Hard
   b. Moderate
   c. Normal

6. How would you describe your smoking habits?
   a. Never smoked
   b. Used to smoke
   c. Currently smoke

7. How would you describe your blood pressure?
   a. It's within the normal range (120/80 or lower)
   b. It's a little high (120/80 to 140/90)
   c. It's very high (140/90 or higher)
   d. I don't know

8. How would your doctor describe your current weight?
   a. I am at a healthy weight
   b. I could stand to lose a few pounds
   c. I should probably lose 10 to 20 pounds
   d. I should lose 30 pounds or more

9. Have you been diagnosed with any of the following diseases? (Check all that apply.)

   a. Heart disease

   b. Stroke

   c. Diabetes

   d. Asthma

   e. Sleep apnea

   f. High blood pressure

   g. High cholesterol

   h. None of the above

10. Do you have a parent or sibling with any of the following diseases? (Check all that apply.)

    a. Heart disease

    b. Stroke

    c. Diabetes

    d. None of the above

Scoring

Please give yourself the corresponding point value for each of your answers:

Question 1: a=0, b=1

Question 2: a=0, b=2

Question 3: a=0, b=1, c=0, d=0

Questions 4 and 5: a=0, b=1, c=4

Questions 6 and 7: a=0, b=3, c=8, d=0

Question 8: a=0, b=1, c=3, d=8

Question 9: a=8, b=8, c= 8, d=2, e=2, f=4, g=4, h=0

Question 10: a=3, b=2, c=4, d=0

Result Categories: <5 points = low risk; 5–7 points = moderate risk; >7 points = high risk

Risk Category Assessments

Low: Your score indicates you are at low risk for diabetes, heart disease, and stroke. Maintaining a healthy weight and not smoking are two of the most important lifestyle choices that you can make to reduce your risk for disease. Be sure to see your physician for regular checkups, because engaging your health care provider can help keep you on the road to a healthy, long life.

Moderate: Your risk for diabetes, heart disease, and stroke is moderate. Risk for disease naturally increases as you age, so you should begin now to address any unhealthy risk factors you have. You can control your disease risk by making healthier choices and getting your risk factors under control.

High: You are at high risk for developing diabetes, heart disease, and stroke. You have some risk factors that need your attention. Unhealthy lifestyle habits can be a large contributor to disease risk, which means there may be things that you can do to reduce your risk. Consult your health care provider to craft a plan to improve your risk factors. Your physician may elect to refer you to local health resources or personally address your risk factors by prescribing appropriate exercise, nutrition, and, if necessary, prescription medication.

To find out more about your modifiable risk and to take the full test, go to biggestloser.com.

Love and Marriage

As we saw on the Season 8 finale when Antoine Dove dropped to one knee and proposed to a radiant Alexandra White, *The Biggest Loser* has been no slouch in the romance department. In fact, more happy marriages have resulted from the show than from any reality dating show! Clearly, getting healthy does open you up to love.

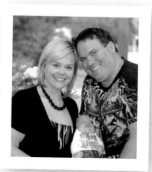

The first *Biggest Loser* couple to marry was Matt Hoover and Suzy Preston from Season 2. Suzy's starting weight was 227 pounds, and Matt's was 339. Today, with two young children, Suzy is working on losing her baby weight and is 175 pounds. Matt is 237 pounds and just completed his first Ironman Triathlon.

"You can tell by seeing us that we've gained some weight back," says Matt. "If you've struggled with weight loss at any time, you know that you have to work at it. We're no different. Our goal now as a family is to change our legacy, so we're not seeing our kids say, 'Oh, my mom and dad were big.' It's an amazing thing to wake up next to your best friend every day."

For Season 7's Nicole Brewer and Damien Gur-ganious, losing weight was important not only for their upcoming marriage but for their future roles as parents. Nicole began the season at 269 pounds, and Damien weighed in at 381. Today, Nicole weighs 155 and Damien weighs 253.

Nicole thinks the wedding was exciting in a way it couldn't have been at her larger size. "I tried on every single wedding gown I wanted, and I fit the sample in the store. Was I in tears or what?" She cried at the sight of Damien in his wedding-day tuxedo. "I was smokin'," says Damien. "That suit is still on fire!"

"But the real story here," says Nicole, "is I wanted to get fit so I could be a healthy mom and have healthy pregnancies. And Damien always said he wanted to be a fit dad, not a fat dad. After the finale, after the wedding, the new thing to look forward to is the rest of our lives. He always says, 'Parenthood next stop'—and I'm ready."

Season 3 castmates Amy Hildreth and Marty Wolff starting dating after their season aired in 2006. In March 2008 they married and today run a health and wellness program in Omaha, Nebraska. And they've added a cub to the Wolff pack—baby Blaine, born in July 2009! Amy says she's using what she learned at the Ranch to lose her baby weight. And Marty adds, "I feel good about myself and it's setting me up for the happiest life that I feel I can live."

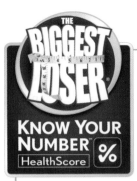

6 Weeks to a Healthier You

The Season 9 contestants are living proof that you can reduce your risk of developing disease in just 6 weeks when you adopt a healthy lifestyle! The chart below lists the results of *The Biggest Loser* Know Your Number HealthScore assessment for several contestants who significantly cut their risk during their first 6 weeks at the Ranch. Each of these contestants took the test when they arrived on campus and retook it throughout their stay. This chart lists their initial (baseline) percentage risk for developing coronary heart disease (CHD) or stroke within 5 years, as well as their odds of developing these diseases and the reduction in their overall risk profile. The results are impressive—and life-changing.

Contestant	5-year risk for CHD or stroke onset at baseline	5-year risk for CHD or stroke onset at Week 6	Odds at Week 1	Odds at Week 6	Percentage of risk reduction
Andrea Hough	41.2%	13.1%	1 in 2	1 in 8	68.3%
Cheryl George	68.2%	27.8%	1 in 1	1 in 4	59.2%
Migdalia Cancel	79.3%	39.2%	1 in 1	1 in 3	50.5%
Sherry Johnston	51.9%	14.1%	1 in 2	1 in 7	72.8%
Stephanie Anderson	37.3%	2.7%	1 in 3	1 in 37	92.7%
SunShine Hampton	42.1%	10.8%	1 in 2	1 in 9	74.5%
Daris George	38.7%	4.7%	1 in 3	1 in 21	87.8%
Koli Palu	67.1%	13.0%	1 in 1	1 in 8	80.6%
Lance Morgan	73.1%	21.6%	1 in 1	1 in 5	70.5%
Sam Poueu	50.9%	5.0%	1 in 2	1 in 20	90.1%

Athletes

Tara Costa is now known as the "machine of Season 7," having won more challenges in her season than any other player in *Biggest Loser* history. Who will ever forget the sight of her pulling that car, coming from behind to win the racetrack challenge? In fact, a fan recently told her that watching Tara pull the car finally inspired her to get off the couch—and lose 50 pounds!

Tara's starting weight was 294 pounds. Today, the Season 7 finalist weighs in at 165. "I was a fat chick and didn't like my life anymore. I was in dire need of help." Tara completed the New York City Marathon in November 2009 and is now planning health fairs and community runs. "I came back to my old environment and wanted to do something. There weren't many road races for runners in my town. For the first one I organized, I thought 200 people would come; 500 people showed up! So many people came up to me and said, 'Because you started losing weight, I just wanted to go along with you.'

"Now I believe in myself," says Tara. "I completely believe in myself. If I put my mind to something, I'll do it. I wanted to get my life back. And I got a *great* life back."

Matt Hoover set his sights on completing an Ironman Triathlon. "I couldn't think of anything harder," he says. "I was intimidated seeing all the

Julie Hadden, Season 4

When I left the Ranch, Dr. Huizenga told me that to maintain my loss, I would have to work out between 1 and 1½ hours 5 or 6 days a week. Sure enough, he was right. I've tried it every which way, and there is no other way around it!

skinny people at the start of the race. But maybe that's why I did it. Sometimes, you need to see a chubby guy taking off and doing it."

After completing the swim and getting 50 miles into the bike ride, he felt queasy and vomited. But he thought back to his *Biggest Loser* Ranch days, just as he always does when he's doing something tough. "I remember before I got on the show, I was lying on the couch with a bag of chips on my gut and thinking, 'I should try to get on that show. I wonder what would happen?' I don't think I was alone. I think a lot of people lie around and think of all the things they could be doing. They don't get up off the couch and go. But that's when you start to see changes."

Matt strived to finish the triathlon in under 17

hours so he could be an official finisher. As he struggled to complete the marathon portion in the dark, he could hear the cheers of onlookers. He missed the cutoff by 3 minutes. "But I crossed that finish line; I never quit. I look back on that race and how it changed me. It made me realize it's not about how much you weigh. It's not about what you've done in your past. It's about what you do. Bodies? They're amazing. I shouldn't have been able to do what I did that day. But my body kept going. There's something about pushing yourself beyond your limits that people need to do once in their lives. They need to take the chance one time to see what they really can do. Once you do it, you're never the same."

Changes

Three years ago, Season 4's Julie Hadden weighed 218 pounds on a 5-foot-1-inch frame. The mother of one son, she wanted to have another child—but after visiting a fertility doctor, she was told she has polycystic ovaries and would need to lose weight to improve her health and her chances of conceiving.

At the Ranch, she says she learned that she was "stronger than she ever thought she could possibly be. What it taught me most of all was that I was worthy to live the life that I dreamed of. I didn't believe it before." Once she returned home health-ier and with a new perspective on life, she and her husband decided that they wanted to adopt, which is what they did.

"I love my life," says Julie. "I have a new life that's going to be well spent and well lived. I changed it. That was the best thing I ever did, getting my life back." Today, she weighs between 128 and 135 pounds.

Vicky Vilcan emerged from her season "the biggest game player who ever walked in this house," according to trainer Bob Harper. After starting Season 6 at 246 pounds, today she weighs 150. "I know who I am, I know who I'm not. I look the way I do now because I'm proud of myself and I made positive changes," she says.

"Before *The Biggest Loser,* I didn't cook meals, didn't think I had the time. I would go pick up

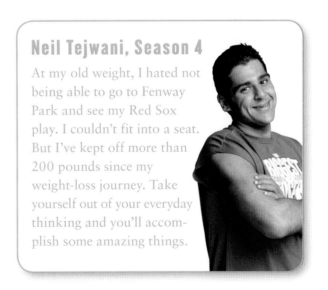

Neil Tejwani, Season 4

At my old weight, I hated not being able to go to Fenway Park and see my Red Sox play. I couldn't fit into a seat. But I've kept off more than 200 pounds since my weight-loss journey. Take yourself out of your everyday thinking and you'll accomplish some amazing things.

chicken nuggets and french fries every single day for the kids. *Now* I know it doesn't take long if you just take a few hours a week to prepare. Once a week, I make a batch of turkey chili. A cup is about 200 calories. It's a nice balance of protein and complex carbs."

Filipe and Sione Fa, the Tongan cousins from Season 7, have taken their healthy lifestyle back to their community. Sione's namesake grandfather died of diabetes when he was in his early 60s and had been blind from the disease the last 5 years of his life.

"If we can inspire someone in our community to make healthier choices," says Filipe, "that's what it's all about. We can't change a whole culture, but we can inspire someone."

"If we can't change tradition," says Sione, "let's help tradition. If we teach our kids to eat healthy, they'll eat healthy. It's up to us. We have that responsibility as parents."

Today, they hold weekly exercise classes. And at traditional luaus, instead of smoking a whole pig, with fatty crackling skin and all, they cook lean pork tenderloins with the same flavorful seasonings.

Filipe started his season at 364 pounds and

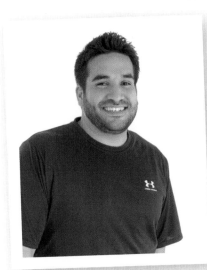

today weighs 242. Sione started at 372 pounds and now weighs 240.

Jackie Evans, who teamed up with her son Dan in Season 5, knew she needed to set a better example for her kids. "Here I was the mom dishing up the fast foods for dinner, and then Dan weighed 310 pounds. His self-esteem was so low," she recalls. "That was just heartbreaking for me. I remember watching him on the Ranch as he blossomed and grew and began to conquer life."

"The most important thing I learned on *The Biggest Loser*," says Dan, "is that there's nothing that can hold me back. I always thought my weight was going to stop me from living a dream. But I found out if there's something I want to do, I can do it if I focus all my effort and attention. I spent a lot of years not living the life I wanted to. Now I'm literally living and seeing my dream happen right in front of me."

"To go from my son not being able to pursue his dreams because he's overweight to being there at the back of room going, 'Look at my son, look at that kid rock his dreams,' it's great," says Jackie.

Before and After

Season 5 champ Ali Vincent clearly remembers hearing that phrase from one of the executive producers of the show during a casting—that she would forever measure her life as "before and after" *The Biggest Loser* show. "He's got to be kidding," she thought to herself. "I'm here to lose weight. This isn't going to be that big of a life change." Boy, was she wrong. Arriving at the ranch with her mom, Bette-Sue Burklund, Ali weighed 234 pounds. Bette-Sue weighed 261. Today, Ali lives at 125 pounds and Bette-Sue at 160.

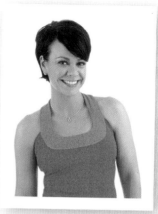

Once a nationally ranked synchronized swimmer, Ali had checked out of all physical activities before going to the Ranch. "I didn't feel worthy to be around people," she says. "But I was tired of being unhappy; I was tired of not feeling good about myself. It had gotten to the point where I felt I was in this big, black hole and didn't know how to get out.

"Now I know I can do whatever I want to," says Ali. "My body no longer holds me back. I know how to go 100 percent now. I know that if I believe it, I can be it."

And what did Bette-Sue figure out? "That I wasn't going to die just because I exerted myself completely," she laughs.

Bill Germanakos, Season 4 Winner

Being in the clinical laboratory business, I knew what all my numbers were. Today I weigh 209 pounds, down from my starting weight of 334 pounds. Eating right and exercising, I've been able to completely reverse all of my "bad numbers." I'm off all my medications. My blood pressure is perfect. My cholesterol count is perfect.

What enables these contestants to reclaim their lives—their marriages, families, jobs, self-esteem, and goals? Quite simply: their healthy bodies. It's a lot easier to be happy, active, and *alive* in a body that supports your dreams instead of holding you back from them. Don't let poor health stop you from living the life you want. Get started now—you're just 6 weeks away from a healthier you!

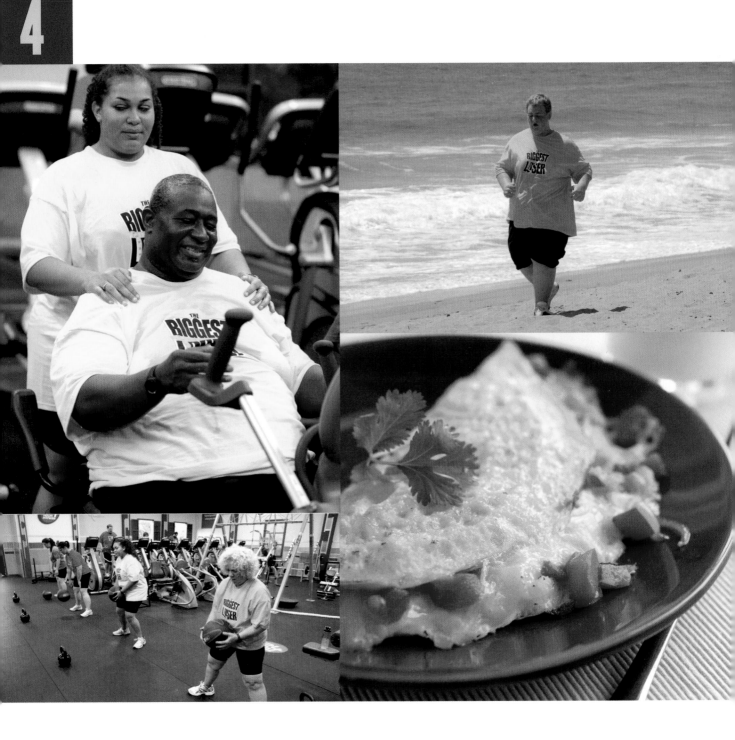

4

Week 1: Prevent and Reverse Diabetes

During the first episode of Season 8, Dr. Robert Huizenga sat down with contestant Sean Algaier to review his medical chart. "I just have one question," Dr. Huizenga said to the 29-year-old Oklahoman. "How can somebody who has more than 300 pounds of fat write on his medical questionnaire, 'no medical problems'?"

Sean, who weighed 444 pounds that first week on the Ranch, replied, "I don't have type 2 diabetes or anything like that."

"Sean," Dr. Huizenga said, "you *do* have type 2 diabetes."

It was a crushing moment for the father of two young children, with another child on the way. He knew he was overweight, but he still thought of himself as relatively healthy. He dreaded breaking the news to his pregnant wife back home. In the end, he didn't have to. After 7 days and a 22-pound weight loss, his blood tests showed that his diabetes was gone.

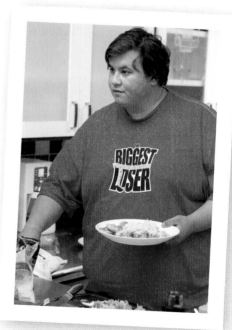

"That week was the most painful 7 days of my life," Sean admits. "But I followed *The Biggest Loser* eating plan, just like all the other contestants, and worked my butt off in that gym. The thing is, type 2 diabetes is completely reversible through diet and exercise. Honestly, after a diagnosis like that, are you really going to look your family in the eye and say you're not willing to do what it takes to avoid an early death? Would I choose a cheeseburger over my family?"

Jenn Widder of Season 5 remembers, "At the Ranch, I was told I was prediabetic. That really,

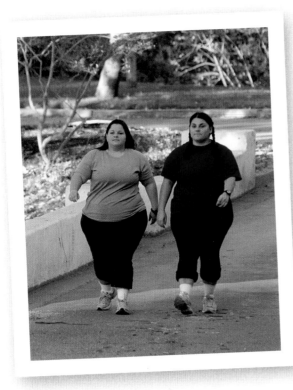

really freaked me out. At the time, I was 22! Diabetes runs in my family, but I thought, 'I am so young, this won't affect me yet.' Boy, was I wrong! But after I lost my first 20 pounds, I was out of the prediabetic zone."

Season 7 finalist Jerry Hayes also provided an early moment of medical drama. After he slumped over in a faint during a workout, his teammate and wife, Estella, watched in horror as medics rushed to his side. "I was afraid I was going to lose him," she says.

Jerry weighed 369 pounds that day on the Ranch. "I had been a couch potato for 25 or 30 years," he says. He had been diagnosed with type 2 diabetes 5 years earlier and was on two medications. He'd been living with gout for 30 years. Today, Jerry weighs 193 pounds and has been medication free for over a year. "Something happened. It started with the show, but something triggered a change," he says.

Now Jerry exercises 6 days a week for 1 to 2 hours a day. "I *like* going to the gym," Jerry says. "Estella and I want people to know that it's never too late to get healthy."

About Diabetes

As many *Biggest Losers* can attest, diabetes is a silent disease that can cause serious health problems, including nerve damage, retinal damage that may lead to blindness, kidney damage, and increased risk of death from heart attack or stroke.

Currently, more than 20 million Americans are living with diabetes. That's 7 percent of the US population! And according to recent projections, as many as 44 million Americans will have diabetes by 2034.

Diabetes is a metabolic disorder—that is, a condition that interferes with your body's ability to properly process the energy (glucose) it gets from the food you eat. Normally, your body converts most of your food into glucose, which then travels through your bloodstream as blood sugar. Your body's cells use that blood sugar to generate the energy they need to work properly. Insulin, a hormone produced by your pancreas, is required to allow the sugar to enter the cells in your muscles, liver, and fat stores—it's the key that unlocks the cells to receive the blood sugar.

But for people with diabetes, that key doesn't work. People with type 1 diabetes, a relatively rare condition that develops early in life, don't produce enough insulin and must supplement the body's own supply.

Type 2 diabetes is far more common, accounting for 90 to 95 percent of all diabetes cases. In a troubling trend, the incidence of type 2 diabetes in the United States has doubled over the past 30 years—not coincidentally, as obesity rates have skyrocketed.

Filipe Fa, Season 7

If I can inspire someone in my community to make healthier choices, that's what it's all about. Diabetes is so common in my community. I'm not trying to change a whole culture; I'm just trying to inspire some of the people in it.

Risk Factors

Being overweight and having a sedentary lifestyle (not getting much exercise) are two of the biggest risk factors for this dangerous disease. Preventing diabetes—or maintaining good control over your blood sugar if you have diabetes—is crucial for living a long, healthy life.

Age is another major risk factor. According to the National Institutes of Health (NIH), only 2.4 percent of people between the ages of 20 and 39 have the condition. Between ages 40 and 59, the number leaps to 10.1 percent. After age 60, prevalence more than doubles, to 21 percent.

Unfortunately, the age profile of people with type 2 diabetes—which used to be referred to as adult-onset diabetes—is changing as a growing number of children and adolescents are being diagnosed. Young people with type 2 diabetes are usually obese and have a strong family history of the disease. In addition, physical inactivity—while a contributor to obesity risk—is also an independent risk factor for type 2 diabetes, regardless of weight.

Daniel Wright, a contestant on both Season 7 and Season 8, was classified with borderline type 2 diabetes and put on medication at the age of 12. "When I was in my junior year of high school, I was classified as full type 2 diabetic, and my medicine dose was increased. I also had to monitor my blood sugar through finger pricking," he says.

After he lost 60 pounds in his first 4 weeks on *The Biggest Loser* ranch, he no longer needed medication of any kind.

And who can forget watching Season 9's Ashley Johnston receive the devastating news from Dr. Huizenga that she was diabetic? "Is it reversible?" asked 27-year-old Ashley, close to tears. Dr. Huizenga reassured her that she could reverse the disease if she started making healthy changes.

"We've been playing around with the most valuable thing we have," said Ashley's teammate and mother, Sherry. "Our lives."

What to Watch For: The Signs of Prediabetes

Type 2 diabetes typically takes time to develop and is often heralded by a condition known as prediabetes. As Season 5's Jenn Widder experienced, prediabetes occurs when your blood glucose is higher than normal but not high enough to warrant a diabetes diagnosis. It's a sign that your body is not responding well to its insulin, a situation that experts call insulin resistance. According to NIH, one in four American adults over the age of 20 had prediabetes in 2007. Most people with prediabetes will develop the full-blown disease within 10 years if they don't take steps to reduce their risk.

Odds are good that you won't notice any symptoms of prediabetes (or possibly even full-fledged diabetes). But if you do notice any of the following symptoms, talk to your doctor about getting tested.

- Increased urination
- Increased thirst
- Fatigue and increased hunger
- Sudden or unintentional weight loss
- Vision problems
- Poor wound healing

Jerry Hayes, Season 7

I feel great. I am off all high blood pressure and diabetes meds. My cholesterol is 104. I believe I have added 20 great years to my life!

You should also talk to your doctor about being tested if diabetes runs in your family, if you have low HDL cholesterol or high triglycerides (a type of blood fat) or high blood pressure, or if you have had gestational diabetes or are a member of an ethnic or racial group at high risk of diabetes. NIH also recommends routine testing for insulin resistance or prediabetes for *all* adults age 45 and older—not just for people who are overweight.

When doctors measure your blood sugar levels, they classify the results according to the type of test you take. Measurements are in milligrams per deciliter of blood (mg/dl). The chart below provides the classifications for blood glucose levels.

Blood Glucose Classifications

Test type	Glucose level	Classification
Fasting glucose: Blood drawn after 8-hour fast	Less than 100 mg/dl	Normal
	100–125 mg/dl	Prediabetes
	126 mg/dl and over	Diabetes
Oral glucose tolerance: Blood drawn 2 hours after fasting overnight and then drinking an extremely sweet liquid in your health care provider's office	Less than 140 mg/dl	Normal
	140–199 mg/dl	"Impaired glucose tolerance" or prediabetes
	200 mg/dl and over	Diabetes

Cheryl George, Season 9

Just feeling better and looking better after a few weeks motivated me for the long term. This is what I want for myself for the rest of my life. I'm not living in a 76-year-old body anymore. Life is too short to sit on the couch. Remember, you are never too old to exercise.

If your blood test indicates that you are at risk of diabetes, here's the good news: Lifestyle changes can have a powerful influence in staving off the disease. In fact, a major NIH study found that people can cut their risk of developing diabetes by 58 percent! Diet and lifestyle changes are essential for diabetes prevention. Even if you already have diabetes, the same strategies can help limit the damage, reverse the disease's progress, and lessen the severity of symptoms.

The Weight-Loss Connection

A Harvard study that tracked the lifestyles of more than 80,000 women (some diabetic, others not) found that excess weight is the single most important predictor of developing type 2 diabetes. Similarly, research shows that losing weight is a powerful weapon against the disease.

Living with Diabetes

Patti Anderson, Season 9

I am 55 years old—the oldest contestant in my season. I believe I represent the average middle-aged woman who has so much—a wonderful family, a great business, terrific friends—but who gives more to others than to herself and, as a result, has neglected her health. I have type 2 diabetes.

I was diagnosed about 20 years ago. It angers me to think that I've wasted the past 20 years and didn't do something to change what was happening to my body. I've been taking medications all these years, but my condition only got worse as I gained weight.

When I arrived at the Ranch, I was on nine medications, and it was an effort to get in and out of my car. Today, I am working out 5 or 6 days per week, eating healthy and satisfying foods, and am down to three medications. I recently ran my first 5-K and have lost 42 pounds since my first weigh-in.

The testing that Dr. Huizenga provided me, along with his vast expertise, has saved my life. I will forever be grateful to him and to everyone at *The Biggest Loser* for giving me the knowledge and tools to become the woman I want to be (inside and out)!

Knowledge is so powerful. When I learned just how sick I was, I knew I would be throwing years away if I didn't change. I want as many healthy years as possible. My father died suddenly when he was my age. I want to live a long, healthy life—and with the help of my family and friends, I will succeed!

I know now that it's okay to concentrate on me and that I can succeed in becoming fit and healthy, no matter how long it's been. It's never too late to start!

Season 7's Ron Morelli, age 55, was affectionately known on the show as "Don Ron" for his agility at gamesmanship. But at a starting weight of 430 pounds, he might have been known as "Mr. Medication." Having lived with type 2 diabetes for 15 years, he was taking insulin plus eight medications for diabetes and other ailments when he arrived at *The Biggest Loser* Ranch.

Today, Ron has lost the weight—and the meds. He is no longer on insulin and takes only one medication each day. What has he gained? "I've gained the fact that I'm going to see my children walk down the aisle," he says. "That I'm going to meet my grandchildren."

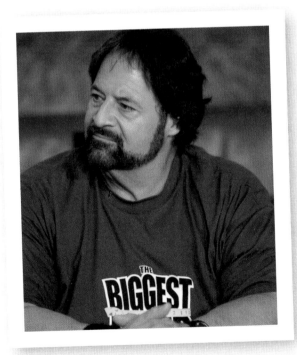

Understand Your GI Bill

Whether or not you're in the military, you should be familiar with the GI—that is, the glycemic index. The GI scale ranks foods by how quickly their carbohydrates turn into glucose. A food's GI and its amount of carbohydrate per serving combine to make up its total glycemic load (GL). Eating the right foods will help you balance your blood sugar and insulin levels throughout the day rather than letting them soar, then crash, over and over again. Keeping your blood sugar levels steady is a key component of weight loss.

At times, you might benefit from food with a high glycemic load—such as before a workout, when you need to fuel your muscles. But in general, it's best to opt for low-GI and low-GL foods. The handy reference chart on the next page provides GI values for common foods. In addition, here are some tips for choosing low-GI and low-GL foods.

- Skip sweet beverages. Sugary beverages—including fruit juice, sugar-laced sports drinks, and soda—have a high glycemic load, and consumption of these drinks is associated with increased risk of diabetes. The results of a Harvard study showed that women who drank one or more sugar-sweetened beverages per day had an 83 percent higher risk of type 2 diabetes compared with women who drank less than one sugar-sweetened beverage per month.

Glycemic Indexes and Loads of Common Foods

Food	Serving size	Glycemic index	Glycemic load
Cornflakes	½ cup	119	13
Potato, baked, without skin	1 medium	85	29
Pretzels	1 ounce	83	18
Rice cakes	3 small	82	4
Banana	1 medium	77	19
Sweet potato, baked, with skin	1 small	77	15
Doughnut, cake	4-inch	76	36
French fries	5 ounces	75	39
Plain bagel	3 ounces; 1 medium	72	36
Popcorn, plain, microwave	1½ cup	72	5
White rice	½ cup	72	15
Parsnips	½ cup	69	7
Sugar	1 tablespoon	68	9
Pineapple, diced	½ cup	66	6
Raisins	2 tablespoons	64	10
Sweet corn, cooked	½ cup	60	10
Brown rice syrup	1 tablespoon	55	12
Honey	1 tablespoon	55	9
Apple, with peel	1 medium	54	9
Orange juice	4 ounces	53	6
Brown rice, cooked	½ cup	50	10
Chickpeas, cooked	½ cup	47	8
Agave nectar	1 tablespoon	46	7
Green grapes	½ cup	46	6
Orange	1 medium	42	6
Pinto beans, cooked	½ cup	39	5
Barley, cooked	½ cup	36	8
Fat-free milk	1 cup	32	4
Bok choy	1 cup	0	0
Cauliflower	½ cup	0	0
Celery	1 medium stalk	0	0
Walnuts	2 tablespoons	0	0

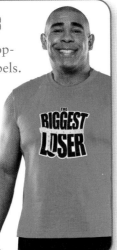

Allen Smith, Season 8

When you're out grocery shopping, pay attention to the labels. Look at what you're putting in your body. Just because it says "low fat" doesn't mean it's low in calories. And it's all about calories. You've got to count those calories! Make sure you're burning off more than you're taking in.

- Eat whole grain carbs instead of simple carbs like white sugar and white flour. The bran and fiber in whole grains make it more difficult for digestive enzymes to break down the starches into glucose—leading to a slower, more moderate increase in blood sugar and insulin and a lower GI. By contrast, white foods such as white bread, mashed potatoes, and bagels have a high GI and GL and cause your blood sugar and insulin levels to spike, which in turn may lead to increased diabetes risk.

- If you have a choice between a starchy vegetable and a vegetable with a low GI, go with the one that won't cause a spike in blood sugar. That's easy to do if you follow *The Biggest Loser* plan, which focuses on high-water, low-starch vegetables.

Get Plenty of Chromium

Chromium is an essential mineral—meaning that our bodies don't produce it, so it's essential we get it from our diet. Chromium helps metabolize fat and carbohydrates. It's also important in insulin metabolism.

Some research has found that chromium supplements may help control blood sugar, but more studies need to be done to demonstrate that chromium is helpful for people with diabetes. A small study reported in 2006 divided 37 people into two groups; one group received a diabetes drug for 6 months, and the other got the drug plus a chromium supplement. Those who took chromium had significantly better insulin sensitivity and glucose control.

The daily recommended intake for chromium is 25 micrograms (mcg) per day, dropping to 20 micrograms after age 50. People taking medications for diabetes should ask their doctor before supplementing with chromium.

Good dietary sources of chromium include:

- Broccoli, cooked, 1 cup: 21.9 mcg
- Whole grain cornmeal, ¼ cup: 10 mcg
- Barley, dry, ¼ cup: 6 mcg
- Edamame, shelled, ½ cup: 2.8 mcg
- Lean flank steak, 4 ounces: 2.7 mcg

Aim for Total Metabolic Health

Your metabolism—the rate at which your body converts fuel into energy—is a natural and constant process. Your basal metabolic rate (BMR), which accounts for 60 to 75 percent of all calories burned in a day, measures the number of calories your body uses for essential functions like breathing and circulating blood. Your BMR isn't easily changed. Three factors affect your BMR:

- **Size:** Larger people burn more calories at rest.
- **Gender:** Men tend to have more muscle mass and less body fat than women and therefore burn more calories.
- **Age:** We tend to lose muscle and gain fat as we grow older, reducing our calorie burn rate.

While you can't change how many calories your body needs to function, you can work to maintain muscle mass—and expend more calories with physical exercise. Additionally, major research is now being conducted by the USDA to study the link between food and the hormones that drive metabolism. To boost metabolic health:

- Get moving—and lift. Incorporate resistance exercise into your workouts to maintain muscle mass. Lifting weights, working with stretchy elastic bands, or doing crunches or ballet barre exercises in which you lift your own body weight all qualify. Check out the week 1 exercise plan starting on page 84 for more ways to incorporate strength training into your fitness regimen.

Power Foods

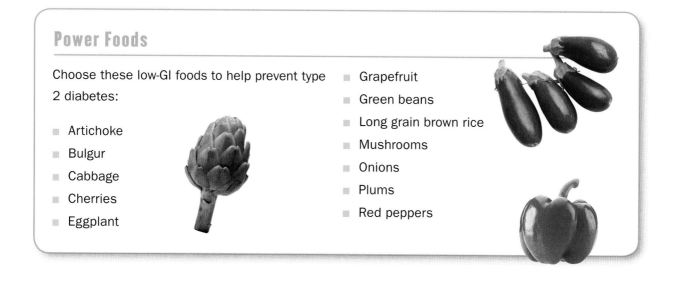

Choose these low-GI foods to help prevent type 2 diabetes:

- Artichoke
- Bulgur
- Cabbage
- Cherries
- Eggplant
- Grapefruit
- Green beans
- Long grain brown rice
- Mushrooms
- Onions
- Plums
- Red peppers

- Feed muscles with lean protein. Aim to get 30 percent of your calories from protein, which will help your body maintain and grow new muscle.

Healthy for the Long Haul

Today, Season 8's Sean Algaier says he's lucky he had a second chance to turn around his health. "If I hadn't lost the weight when I did, I might have died. I'm going to do so many things now. Before my experience with *The Biggest Loser*, I couldn't run or walk with my family. Now I can play with my kids and not be out of breath. I can enjoy that time with them. It's amazing."

You don't need to be a contestant on *The Biggest Loser* to get healthy—and you don't have to be as overweight as Sean was to be at risk of serious diseases such as diabetes. Make sure you know your numbers—have your blood glucose level tested and pay attention to your diet and lifestyle. If you have pounds to lose, use the nutrition guidelines, exercises, and recipes in this book to start getting healthy. "I did most of my work at home, and I still have work to do," says Sean. "Get off the couch. Start right now. You can do this."

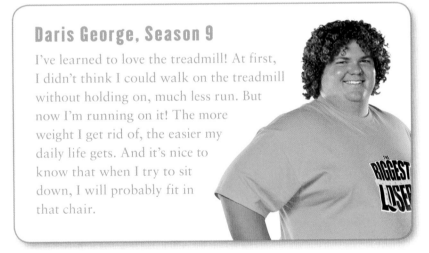

Daris George, Season 9

I've learned to love the treadmill! At first, I didn't think I could walk on the treadmill without holding on, much less run. But now I'm running on it! The more weight I get rid of, the easier my daily life gets. And it's nice to know that when I try to sit down, I will probably fit in that chair.

Week 1 Menu Plan

MONDAY   1,470 calories

Breakfast

Southern Start (page 71)

½ grapefruit

2 ounces Canadian bacon

1 cup fat-free milk

Tea or coffee

Snack

½ turkey sandwich: 1 ounce lean turkey,
2 tomato slices, and 1 teaspoon Dijon
mustard on 1 slice whole grain bread

Lunch

1 serving **Broke Bean Stew** (page 249)

2 cups mixed green salad with 1 tablespoon
low-fat Caesar dressing

1 large apple or ¾ cup cherries

Iced tea

Snack

1 serving **Sunrise Shake** (page 221)

Dinner

6 ounces lean flank steak, grilled

1 cup steamed broccoli with 1 teaspoon minced
garlic and 1 tablespoon toasted slivered
almonds

Sliced tomato salad with ¼ cup sliced green
bell pepper and 1 tablespoon balsamic
vinegar

Green tea or coffee

Ice water

TUESDAY   1,500 calories

Breakfast

1 whole grain toaster waffle with 1 tablespoon
fruit spread

1 whole egg, poached or boiled

1 cup raspberries

1 cup fat-free milk

Coffee or tea

Snack

2 ounces lox or smoked salmon

2 Wasa crackers

Lunch

Roast beef wrap: 3 ounces lean roast beef,
1 tablespoon horseradish, 2 tablespoons
alfalfa sprouts, and 3 thin slices avocado in
La Tortilla Factory whole grain tortilla

1 cup seedless red or green grapes

Ice water or iced tea

Snack

2 low-fat mozzarella cheese sticks and 1 large orange

Dinner

1 serving **Quinoa Tabbouleh with Roast Turkey and Tomatoes** (page 217)

1 cup fat-free lentil soup

¾ cup sliced melon

Coffee or tea

WEDNESDAY   1,530 calories

Breakfast

Jerry and Estella's Veggie Cheese Omelet (page 72)

1 Thomas' whole grain English muffin, toasted

1 tablespoon all-fruit spread

1 cup diced cantaloupe

Green tea or coffee

Snack

1 cup fat-free Greek-style yogurt with ½ cup fresh blueberries and 1 tablespoon ground flaxseed

Lunch

2 servings **Fire-Roasted Tomato Soup** (page 252)

2 cups chopped romaine lettuce with 1 tablespoon low-fat balsamic vinaigrette, 1 chopped hard-boiled egg, 2 ounces crabmeat or baby shrimp, 1 tablespoon

chopped basil, and 1 teaspoon grated Parmesan cheese

1 tangerine

1 cup fat-free milk

Snack

1 ounce sliced turkey

1 pear

Dinner

1 serving **Spicy Seafood Chowder** (page 75)

1 steamed artichoke

2 plums

Sorbet

Green tea or coffee

THURSDAY   1,550 calories

Breakfast

¾ cup Kashi GoLean cereal

½ banana, sliced

1 cup fat-free milk

2 slices turkey bacon

Green tea or coffee

Snack

2 pieces **Cocoa Nut Butter "Truffles"** (page 77)

Lunch

Tuna salad: 3 ounces water-packed tuna (drained), 1 cup steamed green beans, ¼ cup sliced red bell pepper, ¼ cup sliced brown mushrooms, ¼ cup thinly sliced red onion, and 1½ tablespoons low-fat vinaigrette

½ cup sliced strawberries

1 cup fat-free milk

Snack

1 cup steamed edamame

Dinner

1 serving **Sizzling Ginger Pork** (page 78)

½ cup brown rice

½ cup broccoli steamed with ¼ cup sliced yellow or red bell pepper

Green tea or coffee

FRIDAY   1,440 calories

Breakfast

1 slice whole grain bread, toasted

1 poached egg plus 1 poached egg white

½ cup fat-free Greek-style yogurt

½ cup fresh raspberries

1 tablespoon ground flaxseed

Green tea or coffee

Snack

Bye-Bye Blues Smoothie (page 150)

Lunch

Chicken pita: 4 ounces sliced grilled chicken breast, 2 tomato slices, 2 leaves romaine lettuce, ½ roasted red bell pepper, 2 basil

leaves, and 1 tablespoon Dijon mustard on 1 medium whole wheat pita

1 pear

1 cup fat-free milk

Coffee or tea

Snack

2 **Andrea's Roast Beef Rollups** (page 81)

Dinner

4 ounces cod, grilled

8 medium spears asparagus

½ cup cooked barley

¾ cup raspberry sorbet

Green tea or coffee

SATURDAY   1,520 calories

Breakfast

Omelet: 3 egg whites, ¼ cup salsa, and ¼ cup shredded low-fat Cheddar cheese

½ cup fat-free refried beans

1 corn tortilla, warmed

1 cup fat-free milk

1 banana

Green tea or coffee

Snack

4 tablespoons hummus and 8 whole wheat pita chips

Lunch

1 **Mexican Turkey Burger** (page 82), with
1 tablespoon reduced-sugar barbecue sauce,
2 tablespoons fresh salsa, and 3 slices
(1 ounce) fresh avocado on
1 toasted Arnold Sandwich Thin

½ cup diced honeydew melon and ¼ cup sliced
strawberries

1 cup fat-free milk

Iced tea

Snack

5 large shrimp with 2 tablespoons cocktail
sauce

Dinner

4 ounces pork tenderloin, grilled

1 cup cabbage steamed with ½ cup chopped
onion, ½ teaspoon curry powder, and
1 tablespoon cilantro

1 apple, sliced

Green tea or coffee

SUNDAY   1,460 calories

Breakfast

1 egg and 2 egg whites scrambled with
1 teaspoon olive oil and 2 tablespoons grated
low-fat Jack cheese

3 slices turkey bacon

1 cup sliced strawberries

1 cup fat-free milk

Coffee or tea

Snack

8 baked corn tortilla chips

2 tablespoons guacamole

2 tablespoons salsa

Lunch

Grilled chicken Cobb salad: 5 ounces chicken
breast, grilled and diced (without skin); 2 cups
chopped romaine lettuce; 8 cherry tomatoes,
halved; ½ cup sliced cucumber; ½ cup sliced
brown mushrooms; ½ cup diced bell pepper;
and **Avocado Green Goddess Dip or Dressing**
(page 148)

Snack

Banana smoothie: ¾ cup fat-free Greek-style
yogurt, ½ cup fat-free milk, 1 frozen banana,
2 scoops (4 tablespoons) *The Biggest Loser*
vanilla protein powder

Dinner

5 ounces lean roast turkey breast

2 Japanese eggplants, halved, grilled with a
fine mist of olive oil

½ cup brown rice

Cucumber and tomato salad: 1 cup sliced
cucumber; 1 medium tomato, sliced; and
2 tablespoons low-fat balsamic dressing

1 cup cubed honeydew melon or cantaloupe

Green tea or coffee

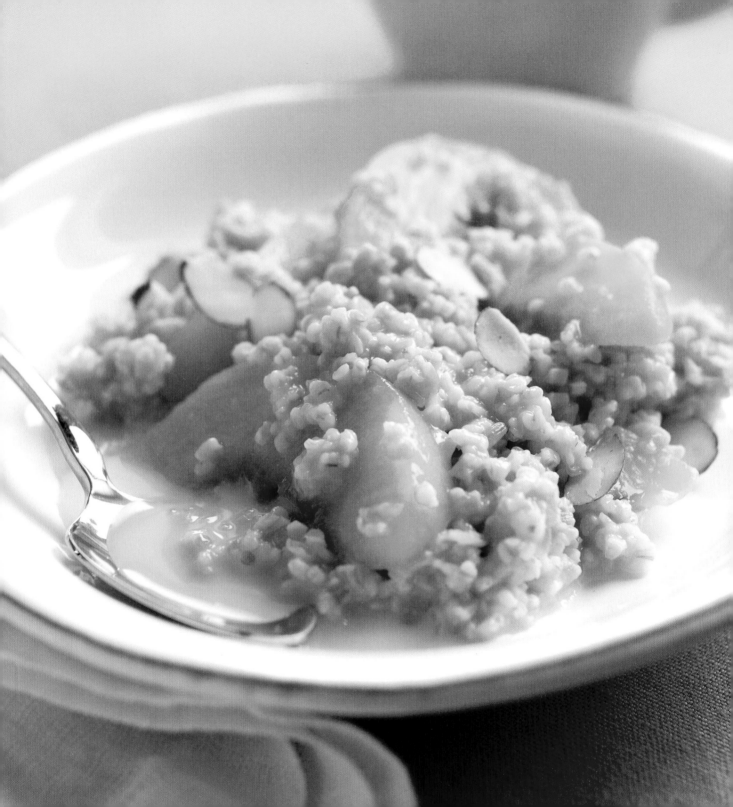

SOUTHERN START

Season 8's Shay Sorrells says, "I just love cereal with sliced peaches and sliced almonds. Frozen fruit makes it possible to enjoy this combo year-round!" Its "peaches and cream" taste will satisfy anyone with a morning sweet tooth.

1 cup cooked steel-cut oats

¼ cup sliced frozen peaches

1 tablespoon slivered almonds

1 teaspoon vanilla extract

¼ cup Almond Breeze unsweetened vanilla almond milk

1 packet Truvia or other natural sweetener

Combine the oats, peaches, almonds, vanilla, almond milk, and sweetener in a cereal bowl and stir well. Microwave for 1 to 2 minutes.

Makes 1 serving

Per serving: 230 calories, 8 g protein, 34 g carbohydrates (5 g sugars), 7 g fat (<1 g saturated), 0 mg cholesterol, 5 g fiber, 45 mg sodium

Estella Hayes, Season 7

My healthy favorites are whole grain oatmeal, whole grain bread, lean pork tenderloin, fish, and protein with fruit at snack time to keep my blood sugar steady.

JERRY AND ESTELLA'S VEGGIE CHEESE OMELET

Like so many people, Season 7 husband-and-wife team Jerry and Estella Hayes love cheese. Here's a delicious way they enjoy it for breakfast. You can increase or decrease the number of eggs or egg whites based on your workout schedule and calorie requirements. Jerry used only egg whites during the final push for weight loss just before the Season 7 finale.

3 large egg whites

1 whole egg

2 tablespoons fat-free milk

¼ cup diced roasted red bell pepper

½ cup diced yellow onion

¼ cup shredded reduced-fat Cheddar or Jack cheese

Chopped cilantro

In a small bowl, whisk together the egg whites, egg, and milk.

Lightly coat a small nonstick skillet with olive oil cooking spray. Heat the skillet over medium-high heat. Add the eggs to the hot pan and cook for a few minutes, until the eggs start to set.

Meanwhile, warm the bell pepper and onion in the microwave for 30 seconds. Spoon the veggies and shredded cheese on top of the egg mixture. Season with your favorite spices and fold in half. Garnish with the cilantro.

Makes 1 serving

Per serving: **225 calories, 22 g protein, 9 g carbohydrates (6 g sugars), 8 g fat (2 g saturated), 215 mg cholesterol, 1 g fiber, 350 mg sodium**

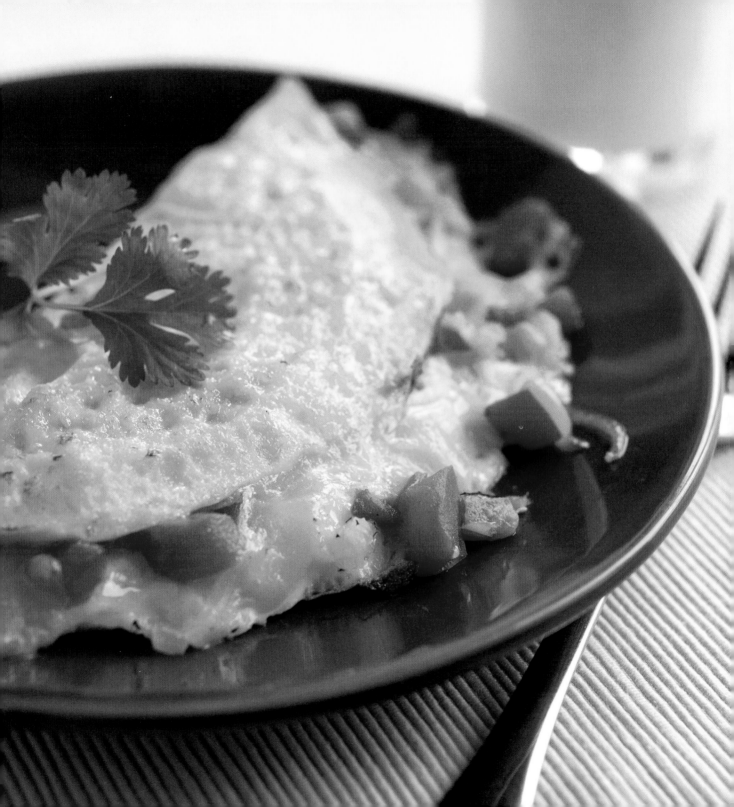

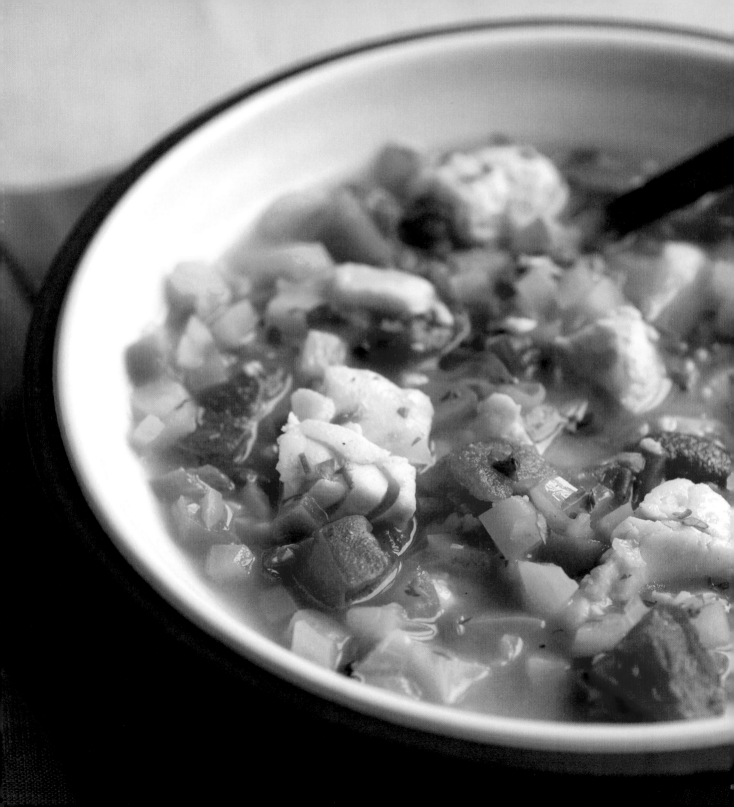

SPICY SEAFOOD CHOWDER

The flavors of this chowder depend on the fish you select—salmon, tilapia, or halibut. You can even use shrimp. Whatever you choose, the intriguing blend of flavors results in a dish that is elegant in its simplicity.

1 tablespoon olive oil

1 cup finely chopped yellow onion

½ cup finely chopped green bell pepper

½ cup finely chopped yellow bell pepper

1 cup diced fire-roasted tomatoes

1½ teaspoons ground coriander

½ teaspoon ground cumin

4 cups fat-free chicken, fish, or vegetable broth

1 pound boneless, skinless fish fillets (salmon, tilapia, halibut, or shrimp), cut into ¾" pieces

2 tablespoons tahini

1 tablespoon grated lemon peel

¼ cup finely chopped cilantro, without stems

In a 3-quart saucepan, heat the oil over medium heat. Add the onion and bell peppers and cook for about 5 minutes, until soft but not browned. Add the tomatoes and cook for 3 minutes longer. Stir in the coriander and cumin and simmer for 1 minute longer.

Carefully pour in the broth and bring the mixture to a boil. Add the fish. When the mixture returns to a boil, reduce the heat to low. Simmer for about 3 minutes, until the fish is cooked through.

Stir in the tahini, lemon peel, and cilantro. Serve immediately.

Makes 4 (1½-cup) servings, or 1½ quarts

Per serving: 240 calories, 27 g protein, 11 g carbohydrates (5 g sugars), 10 g fat (2 g saturated), 35 mg cholesterol, 3 g fiber, 460 mg sodium

Andrea Hough, Season 9

I've come to love fish. I really like swordfish, and it's low in calories. It's delicious sprinkled with lemon-pepper seasoning and served with steamed veggies and a salad.

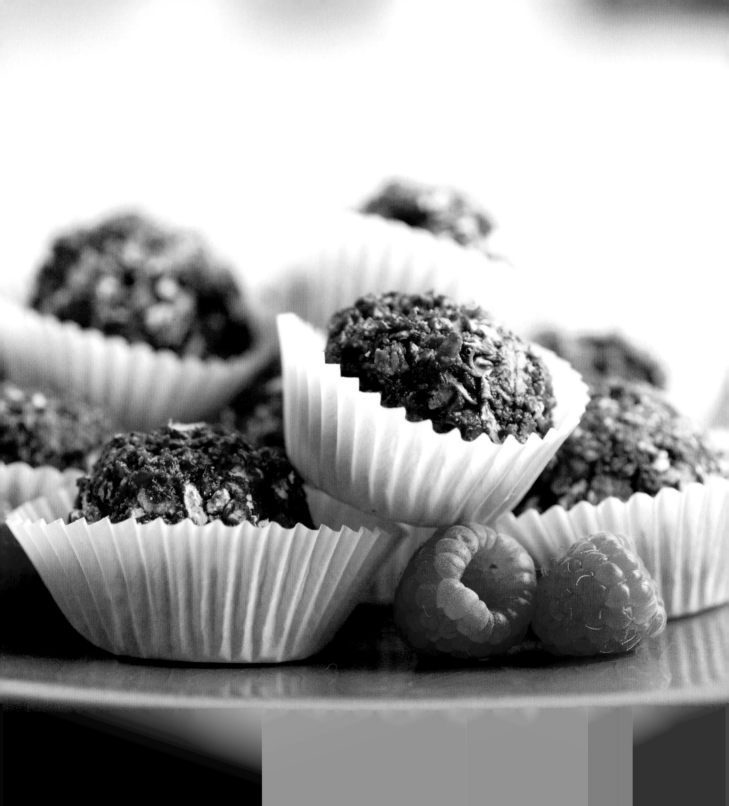

COCOA NUT BUTTER "TRUFFLES"

This delicious snack is high in protein and easy to pack up and take on the go, making it the perfect energy boost before or after the gym. These "truffles" taste like an indulgent dessert but have less than 100 calories each!

1½ cups dry old-fashioned oatmeal

1 cup fat-free powdered milk

3 tablespoons unsweetened cocoa powder

2 scoops (4 tablespoons) *The Biggest Loser* chocolate protein powder

2 tablespoons ground flaxseed

2 packets Truvia or other natural sweetener

½ cup unsweetened vanilla almond milk

¼ cup all natural almond butter or peanut butter

1½ tablespoons vanilla extract

½ cup chopped almonds or walnuts (optional; see note)

In a large bowl, mix the oatmeal, powdered milk, cocoa, protein powder, flaxseed, and sweetener.

In a small bowl, place the almond milk and nut butter. Microwave for 1 minute. Add the vanilla and stir well.

Add the nut butter mixture to the dry ingredients and stir to combine. There will be about 2 cups of mixture. Stir in the nuts, if desired.

Using a 2-tablespoon scoop, form 16 "truffles" and refrigerate until firm. Wrap individually and store in the fridge.

Note: Including the optional ½ cup nuts will increase the calories to about 100 per truffle.

Makes 10 (1-truffle) servings

Per serving: 80 calories, 5 g protein, 10 g carbohydrates (3 g sugars), 3 g fat (0 g saturated), 0 mg cholesterol, 2 g fiber, 50 mg sodium

Sherry Johnston, Season 9

It's vital to learn about the nutrition of foods. Like an Olympic athlete, fuel your body for optimal performance so you can work out the way you need to. I used to be a couch potato, but I've realized how working out makes such a difference in how I feel.

SIZZLING GINGER PORK

Though he usually loved to cook his family's Italian recipes at the Ranch, Season 9's Michael Ventrella concocted this creation one night when I was there cooking with the contestants. It reminded him of a dish at his favorite Chinese restaurant. Michael used chicken, but you can use turkey or, as in this case, lean pork tenderloin.

1 teaspoon sesame, canola, or olive oil

8 ounces lean pork tenderloin (or skinless chicken breast or lean flank steak), diced

½ cup fat-free, low-sodium chicken broth

½ medium red onion, thinly sliced

2 tablespoons finely chopped shallots

2 tablespoons finely chopped ginger

2 tablespoons low-sodium soy sauce

1 tablespoon dark molasses

1 tablespoon Szechuan seasoning (see note)

1 cup cooked wild rice or brown rice

2 cups steamed broccoli

1 teaspoon toasted sesame seeds

2 tablespoons chopped cilantro

In a nonstick skillet, heat the oil over medium-high heat. Add the pork and cook quickly until lightly browned but not fully cooked. Remove the meat from the pan and set aside.

Add half the broth to the skillet and then add the onion, shallots, and ginger. Simmer for a few minutes, until softened. Add the remaining broth and the soy sauce, molasses, and seasoning. Bring the mixture to a simmer and return the meat to the skillet. Simmer for a couple of minutes longer, until the meat is just cooked through. Serve over hot rice with broccoli. Garnish with sesame seeds and cilantro.

Note: Szechuan seasoning usually contains a combination of chile peppers, garlic, ginger, and Chinese spices. You can make your own blend with ½ teaspoon garlic powder, ½ teaspoon red chile flakes, 1 teaspoon ground mustard, and 1 teaspoon ground coriander.

Makes 2 (1¼-cup) servings

Per serving: 360 calories, 34 g protein, 40 g carbohydrates (11 g sugars), 8 g fat (2 g saturated), 75 mg cholesterol, 7 g fiber, 610 mg sodium

Ashley Johnston, Season 9

I've learned to prepare a healthy Asian dish that's quick and easy. I steam a bag of frozen Asian veggies. Then I sauté 4 ounces of chicken or scallops in a nonstick skillet with just one spray of olive oil. I pile the protein on top of the veggies and top it off with ginger-wasabi dressing.

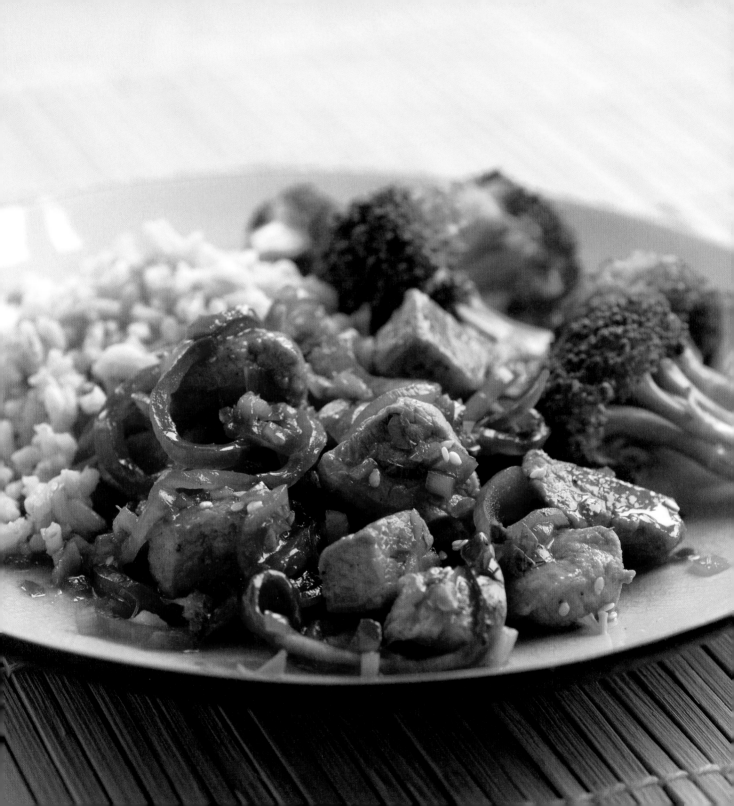

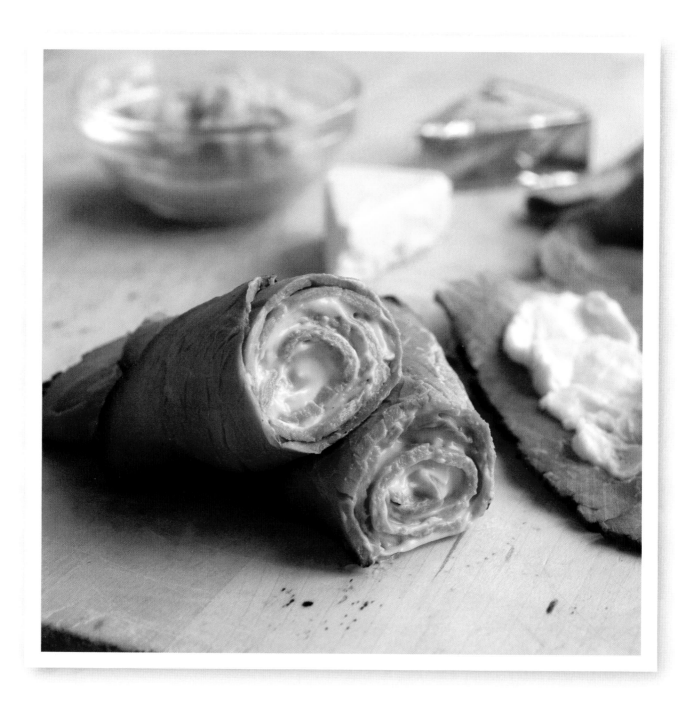

ANDREA'S ROAST BEEF ROLLUPS

This quick and easy high-protein snack was created by Season 9's Andrea Hough for dad and teammate Darrell. Easy to assemble ahead of time, it's a great grab-and-go snack to take to the gym. If you prefer, replace the beef with lean ham or roasted turkey slices.

4 thin slices (½ ounce each) lean roast beef or lean ham or turkey breast

4 teaspoons horseradish

1 wedge Laughing Cow Light French Onion cheese

Spread each slice of beef with 1 teaspoon horseradish. Top with ¼ wedge cheese. Roll up.

Makes 2 (2-rollup) snacks

Per serving: 80 calories, 10 g protein, 2 g carbohydrates (0 g sugars), 4 g fat (2 g saturated), 25 mg cholesterol, 0 g fiber, 150 mg sodium

Cheryl George, Season 9

When you're eating out, divide the food on your plate in half. Either push some of the food to the side or ask the server to put half in a doggie bag right away. I wish restaurants were more responsible when it comes to portion size and calories. But you can make sure they don't determine how much food you put in your mouth.

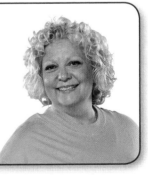

MEXICAN TURKEY BURGERS

These burgers are so tasty, you don't need to add condiments! I like to prepare extra burger mixture, form it into single-serving patties, and freeze. This allows me to prepare a quick lunch or snack on the go. Serving these burgers on whole grain buns kicks up the fiber content.

1 (20-ounce) package extra-lean ground turkey breast

¼ cup chopped cilantro

¼ cup diced red onion

¼ cup diced red bell pepper

⅓ cup diced fresh mushrooms

1 tablespoon Mexican seasoning or fajita seasoning

¼ cup low-fat Mexican-blend cheese

1 teaspoon minced garlic

6 whole grain buns or Arnold Sandwich Thins

6 tablespoons salsa

1½ medium avocados, peeled, pitted, and thinly sliced

6 tablespoons fat-free Greek-style yogurt

In a large mixing bowl, combine the turkey, cilantro, onion, bell pepper, mushrooms, seasoning, cheese, and garlic. There will about 24 ounces (1½ pounds) of mixture, or 4 cups. Divide into 6 (4-ounce) patties.

Grill the burgers for 3 minutes on each side, or until the inside is no longer pink. Serve on whole grain buns or Sandwich Thins topped with salsa, avocado, and yogurt (instead of sour cream).

Makes 6 burgers

Per serving (burger only): **120 calories, 23 g protein, 1 g carbohydrates (0 g sugars), 2 g fat (1 g saturated), 40 mg cholesterol, 0 g fiber, 30 mg sodium**

Sean Algaier, Season 8

My wife marvels at how different I look and feel. She's never known me this small. I'm more driven; I do a lot of housework that I never used to do. You can burn 700 calories in an hour and a half of hard housework! I mopped the floor the other day, and my wife said, "You've never mopped the floor in your life."

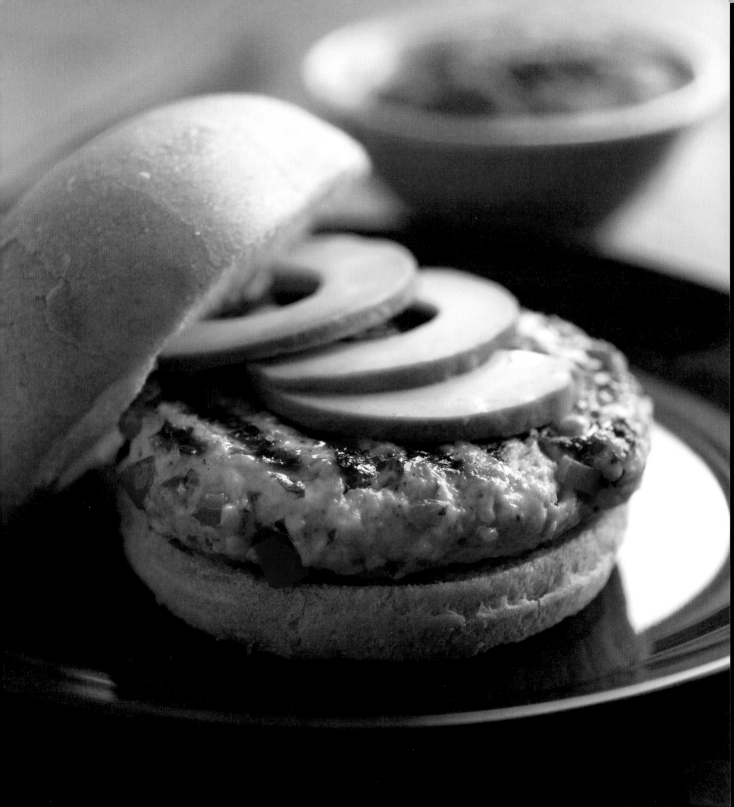

Week 1 Exercises

While any type of moderate exercise is beneficial for diabetes prevention, the exercises in week 1 focus on body-weight training to improve muscle tone and endurance, joint mobility, and flexibility and to create body awareness and a strong foundation.

Body-weight training requires no equipment and can be done anywhere. It increases muscle tone, reduces fat, develops a strong core, and improves range of motion, yet it is less strenuous than heavy weight lifting. *Moderate* exercise is usually recommended for people with metabolic issues and diabetes.

Anyone who embarks on a new fitness program should consult a doctor before exercising, but if you have diabetes or metabolic issues, you should be especially careful. For diabetics, regular activity favorably affects the body's ability to use insulin to control blood glucose levels. However, glucose levels can vary dramatically during exercise, so you should monitor your levels before, during, and after workouts. If you take insulin, you need to adjust your dosage before and after exercise. As always, drink plenty of fluids to stay well hydrated.

Focus: Body-Weight Training
Workout Guidelines

- Warm up for 5 minutes with any basic movement—such as walking, marching in place, or alternating knee lifts—to get your heart rate slightly elevated and to raise your body temperature.
- Begin by completing one set of each exercise and build up to a workout of three complete sets. You can do this by repeating each individual exercise three times or repeating the entire circuit of exercises three times.
- Begin with the basic variation, and work up to intermediate and advanced progressions.
- To add intensity and/or a cardiovascular effect, perform these exercises with no rest in between.
- Follow this workout with a light stretch for the major muscle groups. Most of these exercises actually stretch out the opposing muscle groups, so additional stretching is not mandatory.
- Try this workout 4 to 6 days a week.

LUNGE ROTATION

Begin in a staggered stance with your right leg forward and your left leg back, heel off the floor. Extend your arms in front of you with your hands clasped together at chest level, your shoulders rolled back, and your navel pulled toward your spine. Bend your right knee until your right thigh is parallel to the floor. At the same time, rotate your torso to the right as far as you can, keeping your hands in front of your chest. Straighten your legs and rotate your torso back to the center. Repeat for 1 minute (about 16 to 20 repetitions) and then switch legs and repeat for 1 minute, rotating to the left.

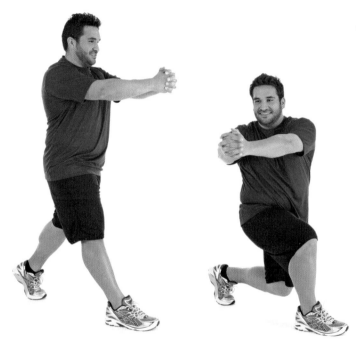

Tips

- Keep the shin of the front leg perpendicular to the floor and don't let your knee go past your toes.
- Squeeze the buttock of the rear leg to press the hip forward and to avoid "dipping" the pelvis.
- Avoid leaning forward or arching back.

Intermediate Progression

Begin with feet together and step forward into the lunge and rotation.

Advanced Progression

Begin standing on one leg with the other knee lifted. Step forward with the raised leg into the lunge and rotation. As you push back to standing, raise the knee again and balance on one leg.

PUSHUP

Begin on your hands and knees with your hands a little wider than shoulder-width apart and your thumbs in line with your chest. Slide your knees back slightly until you create one long line from your knees to the crown of your head, keeping your back neutral and your navel pulled toward your spine. Slowly bend your elbows out to the sides and lower your chest toward the floor, stopping when your upper arms are parallel to the floor. Keep your shoulders rolled back and push back up to the starting position. Do as many as you can for 30 to 60 seconds.

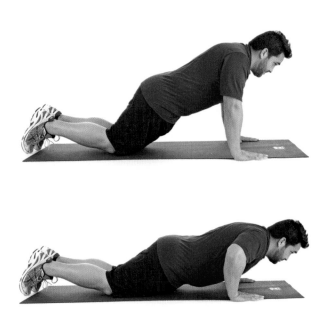

Tips

- Keep your abdominal muscles engaged at all times and don't allow your back to arch.
- Avoid looking at your knees or letting your shoulders elevate toward your ears.
- If you have trouble with the basic pushup, try an incline pushup at a wall or sink. With your legs straight, place your hands a little wider than shoulder-width apart on a wall or sink edge. Follow the guidelines for a regular pushup. Doing an incline pushup changes the weight distribution and makes the exercise a little easier to execute.

Intermediate Progression

Extend one leg so that you're balanced on the knee of one leg and the toes of the other.

Advanced Progression

Extend both legs so that your toes are tucked under and you create one long line from your heels to the crown of your head. You'll be supporting your weight on just your hands and toes.

SQUAT REACH

Stand with your feet shoulder-width apart, toes pointing forward, and your arms by your sides. Keep your chest lifted and your abdominals engaged. Push your hips back as you bend at the hips and knees (as if you were sitting in a chair) until your thighs are parallel to the floor and your hands touch your thighs, calves, or ankles. Push into your heels and return to standing, extending your arms overhead. Keep your spine neutral and your chest lifted the entire time. Repeat for 1 minute.

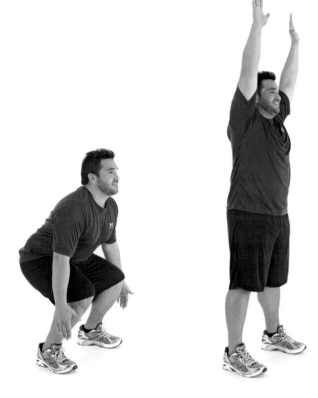

Tips

- Drive through your hips by squeezing your glutes.
- After each squat, try to straighten your arms, biceps by your ears and fingers reaching to the ceiling.
- At the top of the move, pull your shoulders down away from your ears and pull your navel to your spine to keep your back from arching.

Intermediate Progression

As you stand up, lift one knee. Alternate sides.

Advanced Progression

As you lift your right knee on the way up, reach back with your left arm (your right arm is still reaching up) to extend and rotate your torso. Alternate sides.

"W" BACK EXTENSION

Lie facedown on an exercise mat or carpeted surface. Bend your elbows so that your hands are in line with your ears, palms down, about 6 inches away from your head. Gently contract the muscles in your midback, squeezing your shoulder blades together so that your torso, hands, arms, and shoulders come off the floor. Hold for a moment; then return to the starting position. Repeat for 1 minute.

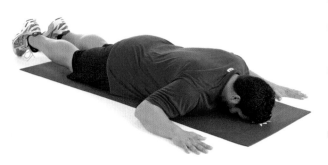

Tips

- Keep your legs straight, parallel, engaged, and on the floor, and pull your navel in.
- Try to keep your hands, elbows, and shoulders in one plane as you squeeze your shoulder blades together and lift.
- Keep your chin tucked down to keep the back of your neck elongated.

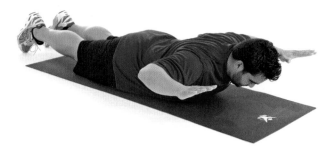

Intermediate Progression

Lift your legs off the floor.

Advanced Progression

While your legs and torso are raised, extend your arms out beyond your head, then pull them back again (simulating a lat pulldown) before lowering your body to the floor.

SINGLE-LEG BRIDGE

Lie on your back on a mat or carpeted surface. Bend your knees and place your feet flat on the floor, feet and knees together, toes pointing straight forward. Bring your left knee in to your chest, holding on to the shin. Squeeze your buttocks and lift your hips off the floor, keeping your left knee pulled in to your chest. Hold for a moment, then release your hips down to the floor. Repeat for 1 minute, then switch legs and repeat.

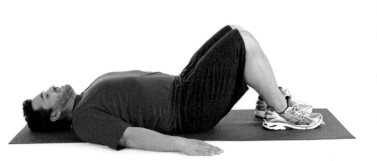

Tips

- Try to relax your shoulders and keep your neck long.
- Keep one foot flat on the floor, and don't allow the knee to splay out.
- Draw your navel in and avoid letting your ribs pop out or your back arch.

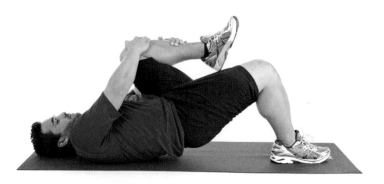

Intermediate Progression

Place your hands on the floor but keep your knee pulled in to your chest (this requires more abdominal activation and control).

Advanced Progression

Extend your non-weight-bearing leg up toward the ceiling for the entire exercise.

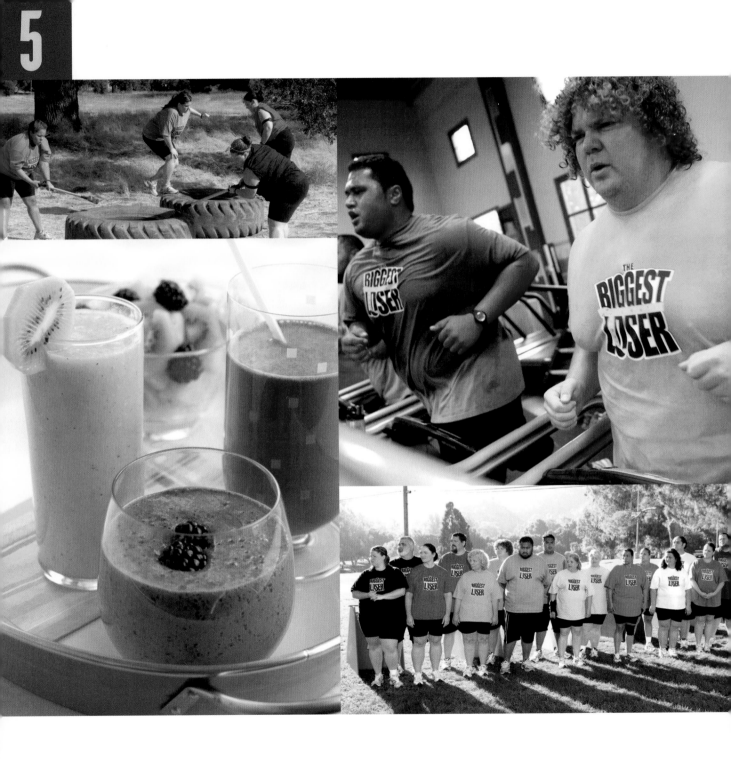

5

Week 2: Heart Smart

"It was one of the most fearful moments of my life." That's how Season 6's Ed Brantley describes the moment he sat down with Dr. Huizenga for his medical consultation at *The Biggest Loser* Ranch. "I realized that my wife Heba's fear that I might have a heart attack before we had a family was valid, and I wanted to change that," he says.

Heba Salama and Ed Brantley came to the Ranch as teammates to change their lives together. The couple wanted to start planning a family and knew they were in no shape to become parents anytime soon. They wanted to lose weight, but before they could do that, they needed to face some hard medical truths.

"Your liver has a type of fat-infiltrated liver disease," Dr. Huizenga told Ed. "When I drew your blood, a cream layer came to the top after we set it overnight."

"You're telling me, but I don't believe it," Ed replied. Dr. Huizenga also informed him that he had prediabetes and high blood pressure.

"I didn't think that much was wrong with you," Heba

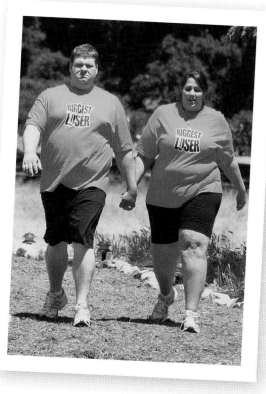

said to her husband in a small, scared voice.

"I didn't either, but here's the reality," Ed replied.

Today, Heba and Ed are both free of illnesses and medications. "We feel less lethargic, more energetic, happier, and revived—like someone woke us up and got us out of a terrible rut!" they say.

"Since we did this together, it has made our marriage healthier in a lot of ways," they continue. "Mentally and physically, we are so lucky to have found a new path that we can follow together and share with our children one day."

With all the pounds, disease, and medications Ed and Heba have lost, what have they gained?

"Our friendships are better, because now we are included in physical activities that we couldn't do previously. We were happy people before, but we never knew we had inner champions and could conquer a more athletic life *and* be good at it. We have gained our lives back, and not just that, but our love for life. Before, it seemed like we were destined to be in those heavy bodies forever."

All of that exercise requires plenty of rest, and Heba says that's another area in which the couple has improved. "Neither of us snores anymore. So we have definitely gained more shut-eye!"

Your Hardworking Heart

Your heart is a life-sustaining muscle roughly the size of your fist. It beats about 100,000 times each day—that's approximately 35 million times a year! It circulates blood throughout your body, transporting the vital nutrients and oxygen your body needs. When your heart can't do its job properly, the result can be an impaired lifestyle or a shortened life span. Your daily habits—including the foods you eat and the amount of exercise you get—play a major role in your heart's health.

What Is Heart Disease?

Heart disease is a general term used to describe various cardiovascular diseases. According to the American Heart Association (AHA), more than 36

Dave Fioravanti, Season 1

I feel *great*. It's been 5 years since I was runner-up for Season 1. I did have very high cholesterol, and now it is around 140, down from 400 preshow! I eat clean every day. It's an automatic lifestyle. I don't diet, and I don't weigh myself. I gauge my weight by my clothes. When I need to, I just take my calories down a bit or work out more.

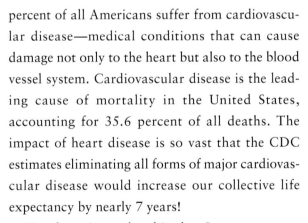

Dina Mercado, Season 8

When I used to eat out, I always ate fajitas sautéed in oil. Now I order the grilled chicken fajita and ask for raw veggies to add to the fajita. It tastes just as good and is nice and crispy and crunchy. And order corn tortillas— no flour!

percent of all Americans suffer from cardiovascular disease—medical conditions that can cause damage not only to the heart but also to the blood vessel system. Cardiovascular disease is the leading cause of mortality in the United States, accounting for 35.6 percent of all deaths. The impact of heart disease is so vast that the CDC estimates eliminating all forms of major cardiovascular disease would increase our collective life expectancy by nearly 7 years!

Your heart is a real multitasker: It routes oxygen-depleted blood from your body to your lungs for recharging, and then it pumps the blood back out to your body through a major blood vessel called the aorta. As oxygen-rich blood exits your heart, some of it is immediately diverted into coronary arteries that fuel the heart muscle itself.

When healthy, your arteries are flexible and allow blood to pass through smoothly. But a condition called atherosclerosis interrupts the flow. Atherosclerosis seems to begin when the thin lining protecting an artery is damaged, allowing cells from the bloodstream to sneak through and enter the artery wall. Substances begin to accumulate, including immune system cells, cholesterol, and calcium. The whole artery stiffens, so it can't expand and contract as it should; the inner passage narrows, too, restricting the flow of blood.

If a coronary artery is damaged, the blood supply to the heart muscle dwindles, which can result in angina, or chest pain. Worse, an accumulation of material in the artery wall can rupture, causing blood to clot and block the flow entirely—resulting in a heart attack and potentially causing permanent damage. Heart attacks and angina can also result in heart failure, a condition in which the heart is unable to pump blood strongly enough.

Risk Factors

The following factors play a role in atherosclerosis and put you at higher risk for heart disease. But don't let the grim statistics daunt you: You have the power to reduce every one of these factors with diet and lifestyle changes.

- **Smoking.** Here's a no-brainer: Quit today. Experts haven't determined exactly how smoking contributes to heart disease, but the toxins released into your blood cause damage to cells in your artery walls, making them less resistant to atherosclerosis.
- **High blood pressure.** Also called hypertension, high blood pressure makes your heart work harder than normal and makes your arteries more likely to develop atherosclerosis. We'll discuss high blood pressure in depth in Chapter 7.
- **Diabetes and metabolic syndrome.** High blood glucose appears to play a role in the development of atherosclerosis and blood vessel disease; people with diabetes are much more likely to develop heart disease than people without it. See Chapter 4 for strategies to keep blood sugar on an even keel.
- **Cholesterol.** This fatty substance actually has many useful functions in the body: It helps insulate nerves, create hormones, and maintain the integrity of each of our cell walls. However, too much cholesterol in your blood ups your risk of coronary artery disease. To travel through the body, cholesterol must be attached to carriers called lipoproteins, which are classified by density.
  - High-density lipoprotein (HDL) is highly desirable; it transports cholesterol to the liver, which disposes of it.

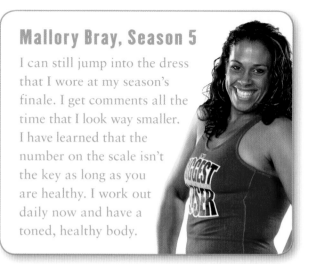

Mallory Bray, Season 5

I can still jump into the dress that I wore at my season's finale. I get comments all the time that I look way smaller. I have learned that the number on the scale isn't the key as long as you are healthy. I work out daily now and have a toned, healthy body.

- By contrast, low-density lipoprotein (LDL) is *least desirable* because it builds up in the walls of your arteries, contributing to plaque.
- Triglycerides are made from either carbohydrates or fat that we eat. Any calories that are not immediately used for energy are converted to triglycerides and then stored in our fat cells.

What to Watch For: Monitoring Cholesterol

The following table provides cholesterol level classifications as calculated by the American Heart Association. Note that measurements are in milligrams per deciliter of blood, or mg/dl.

TOTAL CHOLESTEROL	CLASSIFICATION
Less than 200 mg/dl	Desirable
200–239 mg/dl	Borderline high risk
240 mg/dl or higher	High risk

But those aren't your only important cholesterol numbers. You should also know your LDL and HDL numbers individually. Here's how LDL breaks down.

LDL CHOLESTEROL	CLASSIFICATION
Less than 100 mg/dl	Optimal
100–129 mg/dl	Above optimal
130–159 mg/dl	Borderline high
160–189 mg/dl	High
190 mg/dl or higher	Very high

The HDL criterion is simple: Remember the H's. HDL is highly desirable: You want it above 40 mg/dl, since it protects your health by removing cholesterol from your system so it can't cause damage.

Another way doctors sometimes weigh the risk from your cholesterol is through the cholesterol ratio. You divide your total cholesterol by your HDL. So if your total cholesterol is 180 and your HDL is 35, the ratio is 5.1 to 1. The ideal ratio is 3.5 to 1, so if your total cholesterol is 180, your HDL should be at least 51.

Triglycerides are usually measured at the same time as cholesterol is tested. According to the AHA, your triglyceride results will fall into one of these categories.

TRIGLYCERIDES	CLASSIFICATION
Less than 150 mg/dl	Normal
150–199 mg/dl	Borderline high
200–499 mg/dl	High
500 mg/dl or higher	Very high

The Weight-Loss Connection

The results of a small 2004 study from the Washington University School of Medicine indicated that people who practiced calorie restriction (CR)—eating between 1,112 and 1,958 high-quality, nutrient-dense calories daily—achieved much healthier cholesterol levels than a control group who ate nearly twice as many calories. The people practicing CR had extremely low LDL cholesterol and total cholesterol but high HDL cholesterol. In addition, their blood pressure was "remarkably" low. Their insulin and blood sugar levels came down, too.

Restricting your calorie consumption too much can be dangerous if you're not under a doctor's supervision. But the study underscores a tenet of *The Biggest Loser* eating plan: The *quality* of your calories is just as important as the quantity. The recommendations below will help you combat high cholesterol and the threat of heart disease.

Trim the (Right) Fat

Fat is high in calories. Some types of fat are bad for you. Some fats are actually good for you; they can help increase absorption of key nutrients.

- **Limit your total fat intake.** Fat should account for only 25 percent of your daily calorie budget.
- **Eat less saturated fat.** Saturated fat is solid at room temperature. Examples include butter, cheese, chicken skin, and whole dairy foods.

Reducing consumption of saturated fat is the most important thing you can do to help lower your cholesterol; keep your daily intake of saturated fat to less than 10 percent of your daily calories. To avoid saturated fat:

- Stick with lean meat and poultry and make them even healthier by trimming any visible fat and removing skin from poultry. Use cooking methods that don't require added fat, such as baking, broiling, grilling, poaching, and steaming. Keep meat moist by basting with fat-free broth or a light marinade.
- Always choose low-fat or fat-free dairy prod-

Quick Quiz

Which of the following contestants holds *The Biggest Loser* record for losing 100 pounds the fastest?

A. Mike Morelli, Season 7

B. Erik Chopin, Season 3

C. Rudy Pauls, Season 8

Answer: C. Rudy Pauls lost 100 pounds as of week 7 of his season on *The Biggest Loser*.

Which of the following contestants was the fastest woman to lose 100 pounds on the Ranch?

A. Ali Vincent, Season 5

B. Kristin Steede, Season 7

C. Heba Salama, Season 6

Answer: B. Kristin Steede lost 100 pounds as of week 12 of her season on *The Biggest Loser*.

---

ucts. Use 1 percent or fat-free milk and substitute it for half-and-half or heavy cream in recipes. Opt for fat-free cottage cheese, fat-free ricotta, and low-fat mozzarella.

- **Avoid trans fat.** Trans fat is artificial fat found in hard margarines and vegetable shortenings; cookies, doughnuts, and other baked goods; and foods fried in hydrogenated fat. Here are some ways to avoid trans fat:
  - Carefully read labels of packaged foods. If you see the words "hydrogenated" or "partially hydrogenated," put the package back on the shelf. When you eat processed foods, seek out those using unhydrogenated oils such as canola, sunflower, or olive oil.
  - Steer clear of the drive-thru! Many fried fast foods contain high levels of trans fat . . . not to mention hundreds and hundreds of calories!
- **Choose unsaturated fats.** Many unsaturated fats, classified as monounsaturated or polyunsaturated, can lower your LDL cholesterol and raise your HDL (good) cholesterol. Let healthy sources of unsaturated fats make up the majority of your calories from fat. Monounsaturated fats include olive and canola oils. Fish contains a polyunsaturated fat known as omega-3 fatty acid, which the American Heart Association says can slow down the growth of atherosclerosis and lower triglyceride levels. To boost consumption of good fats:

- Cook with a small amount of liquid vegetable oil, such as olive oil. Use a spray bottle to deliver just the right amount into a nonstick pan.
- Incorporate fish into your everyday dinner menus—but no frying! Choose healthy preparations such as baking, grilling, or broiling.
- Snack on nuts and seeds in moderation. Nut butters, trail mix, and raw nuts pack a powerful energy punch and supply a good dose of unsaturated fat. Keep portion sizes moderate; for example, 14 walnut halves make a 1-ounce serving—that's a small handful.

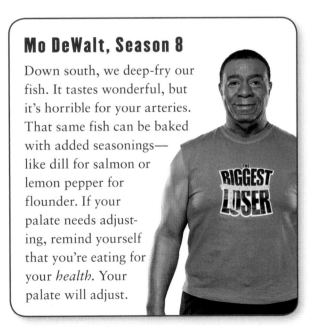

Mo DeWalt, Season 8

Down south, we deep-fry our fish. It tastes wonderful, but it's horrible for your arteries. That same fish can be baked with added seasonings— like dill for salmon or lemon pepper for flounder. If your palate needs adjusting, remind yourself that you're eating for your *health*. Your palate will adjust.

Cut Food Cholesterol

You'll find dietary cholesterol only in animal foods, such as meat, poultry, whole dairy products, and egg yolks. Our livers produce all the cholesterol our bodies really need. Although dietary cholesterol doesn't raise your blood cholesterol level as much as saturated fat does, limit your intake to less than 200 milligrams daily. To cut food cholesterol intake:

- Ditch most of the yolks. Egg whites are an excellent source of protein, but the yolk is pure cholesterol. A few yolks a week are okay in moderation.
- Avoid organ meats such as liver, sweetbreads, and kidney, all of which are rich in cholesterol.

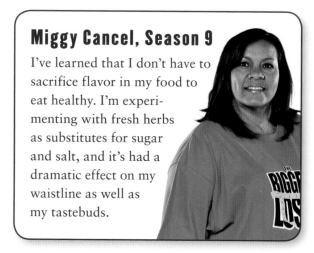

Miggy Cancel, Season 9

I've learned that I don't have to sacrifice flavor in my food to eat healthy. I'm experimenting with fresh herbs as substitutes for sugar and salt, and it's had a dramatic effect on my waistline as well as my tastebuds.

- Limit consumption of shellfish such as calamari, shrimp, and lobster, which are higher in cholesterol than fish is.

Increase Fiber

Fiber is a carbohydrate that your body can't absorb. Found in plant foods, it comes in two types: soluble and insoluble. Soluble fiber dissolves in water and becomes a gel-like substance in your digestive tract. Insoluble fiber doesn't dissolve in water and improves your digestion.

Both types of fiber are beneficial, but soluble fiber is especially important for heart health. Soluble fiber helps trap fat and cholesterol so they can't pass through the wall of your intestine and creep into your bloodstream. NIH recommends that you get at least 5 grams of soluble fiber a day in addition to insoluble fiber; 10 to 25 grams is even better. To add fiber to your diet:

- Eat plenty of fruits, beans, and whole grains to get enough soluble fiber. Good sources of insoluble fiber include cauliflower, brussels sprouts, cabbage, whole wheat breads, and wheat bran.
- Swap low-fiber foods—usually "the white stuff," such as white bread and white rice—for whole grain alternatives.

- Raw vegetables and fresh fruit with skin pack the most fiber punch. Cooking can reduce fiber content in vegetables.
- Increase fiber intake gradually and drink plenty of water to keep your digestive tract moving smoothly.
- Snacks can help boost fiber intake. Choose air-popped popcorn, small servings of dried fruit, or whole grain crackers for a fiber-rich energy boost.

Heart Healthy for Life

When Cathy Skell of Season 7 first met with Dr. Huizenga at *The Biggest Loser* Ranch, he told her she was "pre-everything," including prediabetic. She also had elevated blood pressure, a real concern for Cathy, who has a family history of heart disease.

"My father has artery disease, and my mother had double bypass surgery," she says. "Two days before I left for the Ranch, I was with my father in the hospital. He was having a second stent put in his heart due to severe chest pains."

Cathy worried about leaving her father in such a fragile state. "When I first arrived at the Ranch, I was just waiting for the phone call that he had passed away," remembers Cathy. But, inspired by his daughter and granddaughter's commitment to lose weight, her father decided to get healthy while they were away at the Ranch. "He lost 32 pounds while [teammate and daughter] Kristin and I were at the Ranch," Cathy says proudly. "I feel at times that *The Biggest Loser* has saved his life as well as mine.

"He was even able to fly out for our finale, which was a wonderful gift," Cathy says.

Imagine all the opportunities you could take advantage of with a healthier body . . . activities you could join in, friends you could make, examples you could set, loved ones you could support. Living your healthiest life means living your happiest life. What's stopping you?

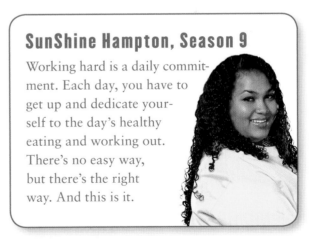

SunShine Hampton, Season 9

Working hard is a daily commitment. Each day, you have to get up and dedicate yourself to the day's healthy eating and working out. There's no easy way, but there's the right way. And this is it.

Week 2 Menu Plan

MONDAY   1,562 calories

Breakfast

Patti's Melt (page 105)

1 cup fresh blueberries

1 cup fat-free milk

Green tea or coffee

Snack

½ whole grain pita with ¼ cup low-fat hummus, 2 tomato slices, and 3 tablespoons alfalfa sprouts

Lunch

1½ cups low-fat black bean soup

2 cups chopped romaine lettuce with 2 tablespoons each diced cucumber, diced bell pepper, and diced tomato and 2 tablespoons low-fat Caesar dressing

1 large peach or pear

Iced tea

Snack

Hawaiian Delight Smoothie (page 106)

Dinner

5 ounces filet mignon, grilled

1 cup green beans and ¼ cup roasted red bell pepper strips

¾ cup wild rice

1 cup fat-free milk

Green tea or coffee

TUESDAY   1,434 calories

Breakfast

1 cup Kashi GoLean cereal or bran cereal

1 cup raspberries

1 cup fat-free milk

1 cup plain, fat-free Greek-style yogurt with 1 packet natural sweetener and ½ teaspoon vanilla extract

Tea or coffee

Snack

2 ounces smoked salmon or lox

2 Wasa rye crackers

Lunch

1 serving **Black-Eyed Peas with Mushrooms** (page 109)

¾ cup cooked barley or brown rice

1 wedge melon

Iced tea or water

Snack

1 medium apple, sliced, with 1 tablespoon almond butter or peanut butter

Dinner

8 medium shrimp grilled with 1 teaspoon olive oil and 1 teaspoon minced garlic

1½ cups steamed broccoli

1 large tomato, sliced, with 1 tablespoon chopped basil and 1 tablespoon balsamic vinegar

1 cup fat-free milk

WEDNESDAY   1,580 calories

Breakfast

1 cup cooked steel-cut oatmeal

¾ cup fat-free milk or almond milk

¾ cup fresh blueberries

1 tablespoon slivered almonds

2 hard-boiled eggs

Green tea or coffee

Snack

¾ cup fat-free ricotta cheese with ⅓ cup cherries or blueberries and 1 tablespoon chopped pecans

Lunch

1 cup whole grain pasta tossed with ⅓ cup crabmeat or baby shrimp, ½ cup diced tomato or fire-roasted tomato, 1 tablespoon chopped basil, and 1 teaspoon grated Parmesan cheese

1 cup red or green grapes

Iced tea

Snack

½ turkey sandwich: 2 ounces lean turkey, 1 teaspoon Dijon mustard, 3 slices avocado, and 2 slices tomato on 1 slice whole grain bread

1 cup fat-free milk

Dinner

1 cup miso soup

4 ounces wild salmon, grilled

½ cup cooked wild rice

3 cups baby spinach, steamed

Green tea

THURSDAY   1,510 calories

Breakfast

3 **Egg White Bites** (page 111)

3 links (3½ ounces) lean Italian turkey sausage

½ banana

1 cup fat-free milk

Green tea or coffee

Banana Fudge Smoothie (page 150)

Lunch

1 cup tuna salad: 4 ounces water-packed tuna, drained; 2 tablespoons low-fat Caesar dressing; 2 tablespoons minced onion; 2 tablespoons minced celery; 1 tablespoon chopped parsley; and 1 chopped hard-boiled egg

1 cup low-fat vegetable soup

1 cup fat-free milk

Snack

4 whole grain crackers with ¼ cup hummus

Dinner

1 serving **Moroccan Pork Stew with Baby Artichokes and Dried Fruit** (page 112)

½ cup cooked brown rice

½ cup fruit sorbet

Green tea or coffee

FRIDAY   1,440 calories

Breakfast

½ large pink grapefruit

Omelet: 3 egg whites and 1 egg, ¼ cup shredded low-fat Cheddar cheese, 2 tablespoons minced onion, 2 tablespoons

salsa, 2 tablespoons fat-free refried beans, 3 thin slices avocado, and 1 tablespoon chopped cilantro

1 toasted whole grain English muffin

Green tea or coffee

Snack

16 raw almonds

1 large orange

Lunch

Grilled ham and cheese sandwich: 3 ounces lean, low-sodium deli ham; 1 slice low-fat provolone cheese; 1 teaspoon Dijon mustard; and 2 slices whole grain bread

2 cups mixed salad greens with 1 tablespoon low-fat vinaigrette

1 cup berries

Iced tea or water

Snack

¾ cup fat-free or low-fat frozen yogurt

Dinner

1 serving **Tortilla-Free Burrito** (page 211)

1 cup gazpacho

8 baked corn tortilla chips

1 cup fat-free milk

SATURDAY   1,540 calories

Breakfast

1 low-fat bran muffin

1 cup fresh blueberries

1 cup fat-free milk

1 hard-boiled egg

Snack

1 stick low-fat Cheddar cheese

1 small apple

Lunch

Sweet Pepper–Chicken Sandwich (page 114)

Lentil salad: ½ cup cooked lentils with
2 tablespoons minced onion, 1 tablespoon low-
fat dressing, and 1 tablespoon chopped basil

2 plums or 1 cup sliced strawberries

1 cup fat-free milk

Snack

½ cup fat-free vanilla yogurt with 2 teaspoons
ground flaxseed

Dinner

Sione's Pepperoni Pita Pizza (page 116)

2 cups mixed green salad with 2 slices tomato,
¼ cup sliced cucumber, and
1 tablespoon low-fat vinaigrette

SUNDAY   1,535 calories

Breakfast

French toast made with 1 egg and 1 slice whole
grain bread

2 tablespoons fruit spread

1 ounce Canadian bacon

½ grapefruit

1 cup fat-free milk

Snack

1 cup edamame

Lunch

Grilled chicken Cobb salad: 5 ounces grilled
chicken breast, diced (without skin); 2 cups
chopped romaine lettuce; 8 cherry tomatoes,
halved; ½ cup sliced cucumber; ½ cup sliced
brown mushrooms; ½ cup diced bell pepper; and
Avocado Green Goddess Dressing (page 148)

Snack

⅓ cup guacamole and 12 baked corn chips

Dinner

1 serving **Cheesy Stuffed Chicken Breast** (page
255)

1 cup steamed brussels sprouts with
2 tablespoons (2 slices) crumbled turkey bacon

1 cup steamed cauliflower

½ cup fresh berries

Green tea or coffee

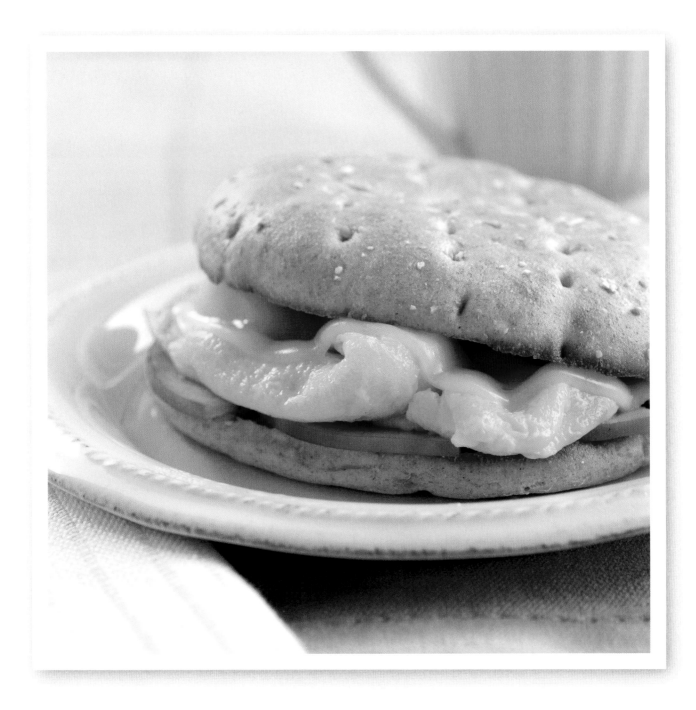

PATTI'S MELT

Season 9's Patti Anderson says, "I made these yummy melts for me and [teammate] Stephanie before walking the Presidential Mile on the Ranch." This low-cal version of a classic breakfast sandwich won't ruin your calorie budget—but it will give you the protein and fiber to start your day off right!

1 slice whole grain Oroweat bread or 1 Arnold Sandwich Thin

2 egg whites or 1 large egg

1 ounce lean, low-sodium deli ham or Canadian bacon

Horseradish or mustard (optional)

1 slice low-fat mozzarella or provolone cheese

Toast the bread. Meanwhile, in a nonstick skillet coated with cooking spray, cook the egg whites or egg. Remove the egg from the pan and set aside. Warm the ham in the same pan for a minute or two over low heat. Spread the horseradish or mustard on the toast, if desired. Place the ham and eggs on the hot toast and top with the cheese. Place under a broiler or in a toaster oven for 20 to 30 seconds to melt the cheese.

Cut in half and serve immediately.

Makes 1 serving

Per serving: 230 calories, 26 g protein, 22 g carbohydrates (3 g sugars), 6 g fat (2 g saturated), 25 mg cholesterol, 5 g fiber, 710 mg sodium

HAWAIIAN DELIGHT SMOOTHIE

This sweet and refreshing protein drink is perfect for postworkout recovery and refueling.

1 scoop (4 tablespoons) *The Biggest Loser* raspberry protein powder

½ cup orange juice

1 cup ice

1 kiwifruit, peeled and sliced

1 cup diced pineapple

1 tablespoon shredded coconut

Combine the protein powder, juice, ice, kiwi, pineapple, and coconut in a blender or food processor. Blend or process until smooth. Pour the smoothie into a glass and serve immediately.

Makes 1 smoothie

Per serving: **260 calories, 9 g protein, 53 g carbohydrates (33 g sugars), 5 g fat (3 g saturated), 0 mg cholesterol, 11 g fiber, 60 mg sodium**

Antoine Dove, Season 8

I try to eat a lot of foods that are low in sugar and sodium and that aren't full of saturated fat. If I am eating foods that contain fat, I'm very careful that it's good fat. I like combining almonds with fruit for a healthy snack.

Hawaiian Delight Smoothie, *top left*, Banana Fudge Smoothie, *top right* (recipe on page 150), and Bye-Bye Blues Smoothie, *in front* (recipe on page 150).

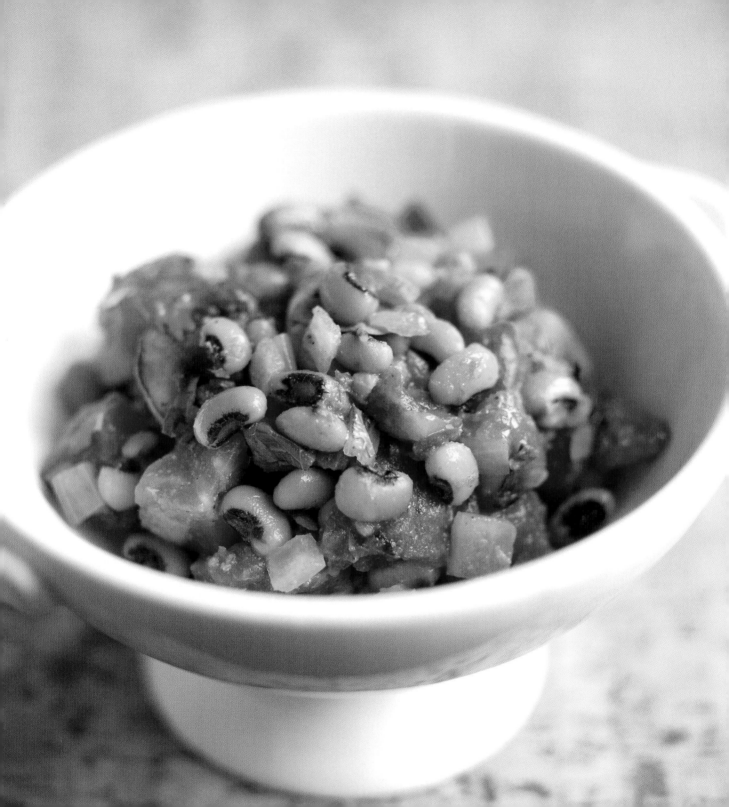

BLACK-EYED PEAS WITH MUSHROOMS

This flavorful vegetarian dish is high in protein, fiber, and flavor. It was inspired by my favorite Indian restaurant near my home in California. Feel free to substitute your favorite beans (or even lentils!). It is delicious when served with brown rice.

3 teaspoons olive oil

1 cup chopped onion

1 tablespoon chopped garlic

1½ cups (14½-ounce can) diced fire-roasted tomatoes (see note)

1 teaspoon ground coriander

1 teaspoon curry powder

1 teaspoon ground cumin

½ teaspoon ground turmeric

½ teaspoon red chile flakes (optional)

1½ cups cooked black-eyed peas, lentils, or beans (black, red, white, or pinto); or 1 (16-ounce) can cooked beans, rinsed and drained

3 cups sliced mushrooms (brown, white, cremini, or shiitake)

¼ cup roughly chopped cilantro

Salt-free seasoning

Ground black pepper

In a large nonstick skillet, heat 1 teaspoon of the oil over medium-high heat. Add the onion and cook for 5 minutes, until softened but not browned. Add the garlic and cook for 1 minute longer, but do not brown the garlic.

Add the tomatoes, coriander, curry, cumin, turmeric, and chile flakes (if desired) and simmer for 5 minutes. Add the beans and simmer for 5 minutes longer. Transfer to a 3- or 4-quart saucepan and keep warm.

In a clean skillet, add the remaining 2 teaspoons oil and heat over medium-high heat. Add the mushrooms and cook for about 4 minutes, until the mushrooms are just cooked and have lost their water. Add the mushrooms to the bean mixture and stir in the cilantro. Season to taste with salt-free seasoning and black pepper.

Note: You can replace 1½ cups fire-roasted tomatoes with 1½ cups chopped, seeded fresh tomatoes or 1½ cups tomato sauce.

Makes 4 (1-cup) servings

Per serving: **200 calories, 10 g protein, 31 g carbohydrates (9 g sugars), 5 g fat (< 1 g saturated), 0 mg cholesterol, 8 g fiber, 240 mg sodium**

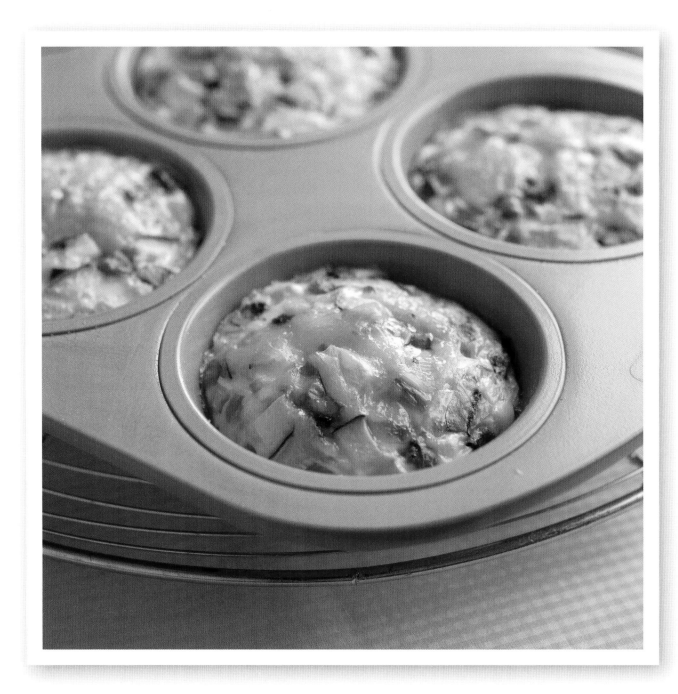

EGG WHITE BITES

Season 3's Jen Eisenbarth and her family enjoy the versatility of this recipe as well as the ease of preparation. I love these for breakfast and usually make two pans so that I have leftovers. Sometimes I make a Mexican variation using cooked ground turkey, red bell peppers, onion, cilantro, and a dash of Mrs. Dash Fiesta Lime seasoning. Once I remove the bites from the pan, I add a tablespoon of salsa and a sliver of avocado. Get creative and invent your own favorite bites!

2   cups grated or finely chopped vegetables (carrots, yellow squash or zucchini, onion, asparagus, mushrooms, bell peppers, spinach)

18 egg whites, or 2¼ cups egg whites or egg substitute

Salt-free seasoning

Ground black pepper

¼   cup grated low-fat Cheddar, Jack, or mozzarella cheese

Position a rack in the center of the oven and preheat the oven to 350°F. Lightly coat two 6-cup muffin pans with olive oil cooking spray.

Spray a nonstick skillet with cooking spray and cook the vegetables briefly, until they reach the desired crispness or tenderness.

Place a small nest of vegetables in the bottom of each muffin cup, then fill the cups ¾ full with egg whites. Add salt-free seasoning, black pepper, and other seasoning, as desired. Sprinkle a small amount of cheese over each cup.

Bake the eggs for about 10 minutes, until they are just set. Cool in the pans.

Makes 12 (1-bite) servings

Per serving: **40 calories, 6 g protein, 3 g carbohydrates (3 g sugars), < 1 g fat (0 g saturated), 10 mg cholesterol, 1 g fiber, 110 mg sodium**

Danny Cahill, Season 8 Winner

The one thing that amazes me is egg whites. I used to eat just eggs. Now I eat a whole egg but add two egg whites to it. That cuts fat and calories and ups the protein. In general, the foods we eat at the Ranch—fresh, whole foods—are so filling that I was surprisingly never hungry.

MOROCCAN PORK STEW WITH BABY ARTICHOKES AND DRIED FRUIT

Sweet spices flavor this sumptuous pork stew. You can substitute chicken or turkey breast for the pork, if you prefer. Serve with a tomato salad and steamed bulgur or brown rice for a delicious meal.

1 pound lean, boneless pork tenderloin

1 teaspoon olive oil

1 large onion, chopped

3 cups fat-free, low-sodium chicken or vegetable broth

1 teaspoon saffron threads, crumbled

½ teaspoon salt

1 medium carrot, cut into ¼" dice

¼ cup diced celery

1½ teaspoons ground ginger

¾ teaspoon ground cinnamon

1 cup pitted prunes, cut into slivers

1 (9-ounce) package frozen artichoke hearts, thawed and cut in quarters lengthwise (see note)

¼ cup chopped cilantro, without stems

Cut the pork into 1" pieces. In a 3-quart nonstick saucepan, heat the oil over medium-high heat until hot but not smoking. Add the onion and cook until softened, stirring to keep from browning.

Stir in the broth, saffron, and salt and bring to a boil. Reduce the heat to low. Add the carrot and celery; simmer, covered, for about 2 minutes.

Add the ginger, cinnamon, prunes, and artichoke hearts and simmer until the vegetables and fruits are nearly tender, about 2 minutes.

Add the pork pieces to the stew and stir in the cilantro. Simmer, uncovered, stirring occasionally, for 6 to 8 minutes, or until the pork is just cooked.

Note: You may use a drained 9-ounce jar of water-packed artichoke hearts. Because they are already cooked, add them at the end, *after* the pork is cooked.

Makes 4 (1½-cup) servings

Per serving: 300 calories, 28 g protein, 39 g carbohydrates (13 g sugars), 6 g fat (2 g saturated), 75 mg cholesterol, 8 g fiber, 375 mg sodium

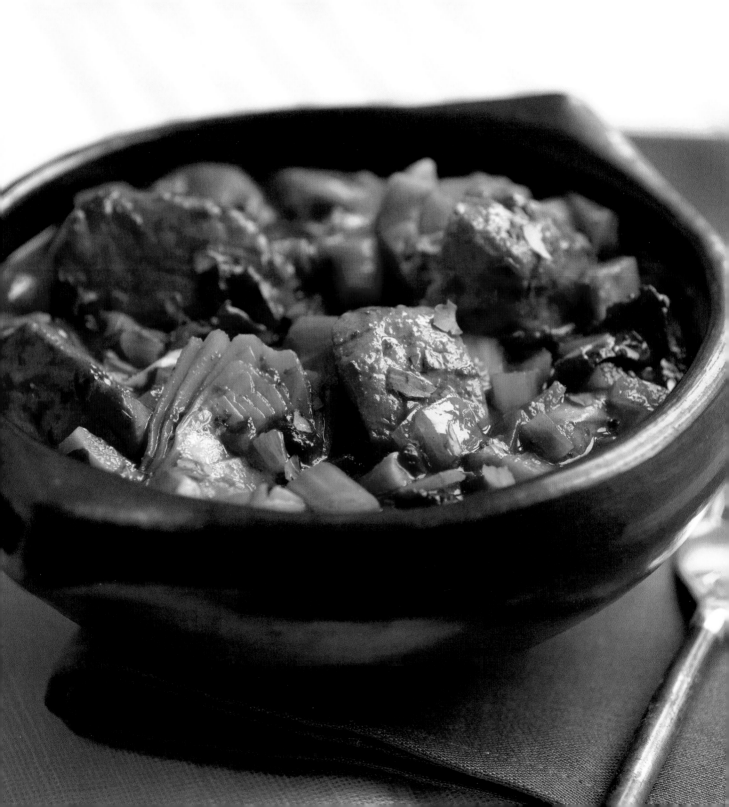

SWEET PEPPER–CHICKEN SANDWICH

Season 7's Estella Hayes and I invented this recipe one day at the Ranch when we were bored with a plain chicken sandwich. The addition of bell peppers gives this sandwich added flavor, and the sprouted grain bread lends a great texture.

1 tablespoon yellow or spicy mustard

2 slices Trader Joe's or other brand sprouted whole grain bread, toasted

1 large leaf romaine lettuce

3 ounces lean, low-sodium sliced chicken breast

½ roasted red bell pepper, cut in strips

¼ cup shredded reduced-fat Mexican four-cheese blend

Spread the mustard on 1 piece of toast. Top with the lettuce, chicken, and bell pepper, ending with the cheese.

Place the half sandwich under a broiler or in a toaster oven for 20 to 30 seconds, until the cheese melts. Top with the second piece of toast. Cut in half. Serve immediately.

Makes 1 sandwich

Per serving: 310 calories, 31 g protein, 30 g carbohydrates (3 g sugars), 7 g fat (3 g saturated), 65 mg cholesterol, 6 g fiber, 1,380 mg sodium

Pete Thomas, Season 2

Learning to eat healthy is about modification, not starvation. Take some initiative. Look at your grocery store circulars and find out when the boneless, skinless chicken breasts are on sale, and stock up!

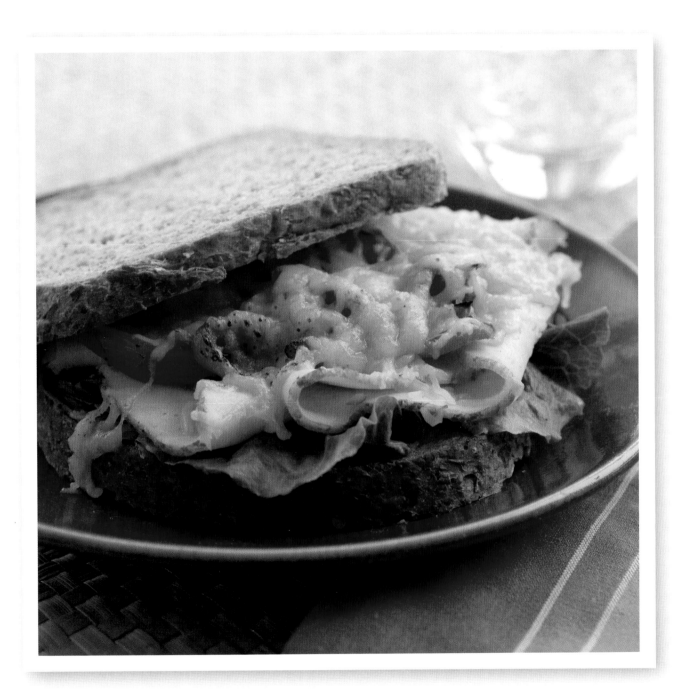

SIONE'S PEPPERONI PITA PIZZA

Season 7's Sione Fa says of this delicious mini-pizza, "We are a pizza family, and my kids can't even tell the difference with this healthier version. The kids make their own pizzas. Not only do they love doing it, but my wife and I love it that we now eat healthy as a family and still enjoy our favorite foods."

⅛ cup low-fat marinara or tomato-basil sauce

1 medium whole grain pita (about 5" diameter)

⅛ cup shredded fat-free or low-fat mozzarella cheese (see note)

8 slices (½ ounce total) lean turkey pepperoni

Fresh basil

Spread the sauce on top of the pita. Sprinkle the cheese over the sauce. Distribute the pepperoni slices on top of the pizza.

Bake in a toaster oven until the cheese has melted. Garnish with fresh basil.

Note: Using low-fat mozzarella cheese will increase the calories to 200 and the grams of fat to 6.

Makes 1 (5") pizza

Per serving: 190 calories, 14 g protein, 26 g carbohydrates (1 g sugars), 4 g fat (1 g saturated), 20 mg cholesterol, 3 g fiber, 650 mg sodium

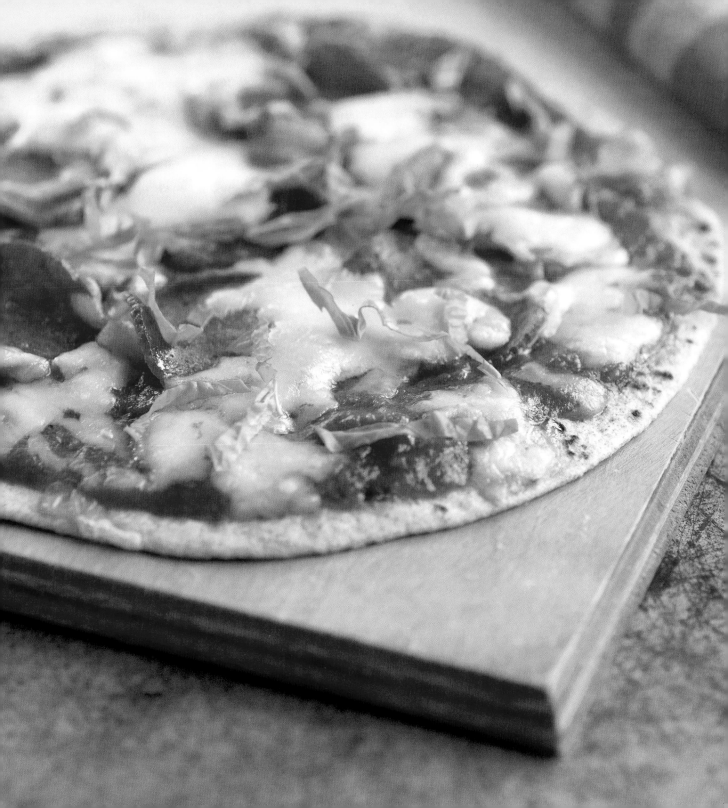

Week 2 Exercises

As one of the key risk factors for cardiovascular disease, a sedentary lifestyle can increase your chance of having a heart attack or stroke. Many studies have established that regular exercise can assist in weight management; reduce body fat; reduce total cholesterol levels, especially the bad variety, in the blood (and even raise good cholesterol!); lower blood pressure; and increase insulin sensitivity/glucose tolerance (see Chapter 4 for more information).

Week 2 focuses on cardiovascular or aerobic training to improve overall health, but especially that of the heart and lungs, which make up the cardiorespiratory system. Benefits of aerobic training include:

- Stronger lungs and heart
- Improved maximum oxygen consumption and lung efficiency
- Increased number of red blood cells that transport oxygen to the muscles
- Lower resting heart rate
- Improved circulation
- Increased metabolism
- Lowered risk of coronary artery disease (CAD), hypertension, cancer, obesity, cognitive decline, and depression

The CDC, the American College of Sports Medicine, and the US Surgeon General recommend that adults participate in 30 or more minutes of moderate-intensity activity on most, and preferably all, days of the week. This includes recreational activities and everyday tasks such as gardening, doing household chores, swimming, playing tennis, cycling, dancing, and walking. If you are new to exercising, accumulating 30 minutes of total exercise over the course of a day (in short 5- to 10-minute bouts) has proven to be beneficial to overall wellness. As you become more fit, increase the frequency (how many days a week), intensity (level of exertion), and/or time (how long you exercise).

If you are just starting out, keep it simple and begin by walking for 10 minutes a day. Aim to do this every day. As you progress, you can build up to 30 minutes. To add variety, try the five exercises on the next few pages to get your heart pumping.

Focus: Aerobic Training
Workout Guidelines

- Warm up for 5 minutes by marching in place or walking.
- Begin with 1 minute of each exercise and repeat the circuit two times. During this second week of the plan, gradually increase to five rounds of the circuit.
- Perform the exercises in the order they are presented. For a higher-intensity workout, try not to rest between exercises.
- Begin with the most basic variation. As you get stronger, work up to the intermediate and advanced progressions.
- Follow up this cardio workout with a gentle stretch for your legs, back, and chest as well as your triceps and shoulders.
- Try this workout 5 or 6 days a week or alternate days with the body-weight exercises from Chapter 4 (3 or 4 days of aerobic training and 2 or 3 days of body-weight exercises).
- As always, check with your doctor for clearance before beginning an exercise program. Stop exercising, rest, and contact your doctor if you experience weakness, dizziness, unexplained weight gain, or swelling and/or pressure or pain in your chest, arm, shoulder, neck, or jaw.

JUMPING JACK

Begin with your feet together and your arms by your sides. Jump and spread your feet out to the sides about 2 to 2½ feet as you lift your arms to the side and over your head. Keep your knees soft and your core engaged and land gently, with your heels on the floor. Immediately jump and pull your feet back in as you bring your arms to your sides. Repeat quickly for 1 minute.

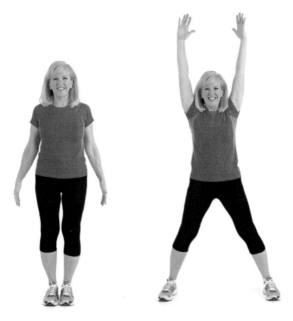

Tips

- Be sure to land gently, with your knees soft, to minimize impact on your spine and knees.
- Don't allow your knees to collapse inward. If this begins to happen, adjust by not jumping out so far.
- Keep your abdominals pulled in and avoid arching your back.
- If jumping jacks are difficult, try simply stepping out to the side, alternating right and left, rather than jumping.

Intermediate Progression

Turn your torso right and left as you jump and spread your feet.

Advanced Progression

Add a deeper squat by bending your knees more as you jump and spread your feet. This will slow the pace down a bit, but you'll get the benefit of stronger leg work.

BURPEE

Stand with your feet at least hip-width apart and your arms by your sides. Squat down by bending your knees, keeping your back straight and abs pulled in. Place your hands on the floor by your feet, then extend one leg back at a time until both legs are straight and you are in a plank (full pushup) position with your shoulders over your hands. Hold for a moment. Reverse the move by bringing each foot toward your hands to return to the squat position, then driving up through your hips to come to standing. Repeat quickly for 1 minute.

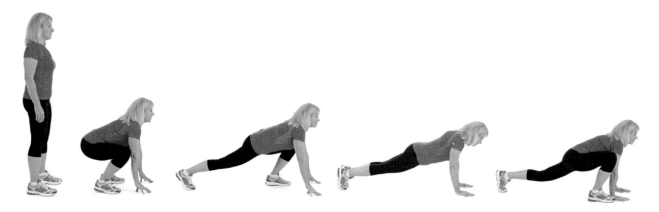

Tips

- If you have restricted movement in your hips, begin with your legs in a wider stance.
- It's very important to focus on keeping your navel pulled toward your spine in the plank position—do not allow your back to arch.
- If you find this move a bit challenging, try using a step platform, a sturdy box, or the bottom step of a staircase to place your body on a greater incline when you're in the plank position.

Intermediate Progression

Replace the step back and the step in with a jump back and a jump in.

Advanced Progression

Do a pushup from the plank position before you return to standing.

HIGH KNEES

Stand with your feet under your hips and your arms by your sides. Start marching in place and progress to a light jog in place, allowing your arms to swing naturally by your sides. Keeping your abdominals pulled in tight, lean back slightly and begin to lift your knees high in front of you. Continue for 1 minute.

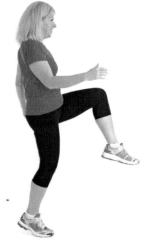

Tips

- Keep your chest lifted and your neck relaxed.
- Stay light on your feet by thinking of lifting up, rather than pounding into your legs.
- If high knees are too intense, return to the march—or jog in place.

Intermediate Progression

Increase speed and/or increase range of motion by bringing your knees higher.

Advanced Progression

Extend your arms overhead.

SKATER

Stand with your feet together and your arms by your sides. Step one leg out to the side in as wide a stance as possible. With your right (front) foot, step diagonally to the left side, leaving your back (left) leg bent at the knee. Allow your body to rotate slightly toward the stepping leg and your arms to move naturally. Pick up the tempo and increase the distance of your steps. Continue for 1 minute.

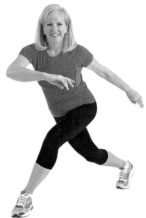

Tips

- To allow for greater range of motion, keep your knees bent as you increase speed.
- Allow your torso to hinge forward slightly as the width of your steps increases. Keep your abdominals pulled in to protect your lower back.
- Maintain proper alignment by keeping the knee of the stepping leg over the ankle.

Intermediate Progression

Increase speed and change the step to a small leap, landing gently with knees bent.

Advanced Progression

Keep your back foot off the floor as you leap from side to side.

MOUNTAIN CLIMBER

Begin in a plank (full pushup) position with your shoulders over your hands and your legs fully extended. Pull one knee in toward your chest with your toes on the floor. (It looks like a sprinter's take-off position.) In one clean motion, switch legs, keeping your upper torso still. Repeat quickly for 1 minute.

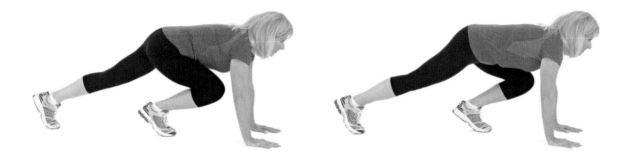

Tips

- Keep the proper shoulder-over-hand alignment so that you safely use your arm, chest, and back muscles to support your upper body.
- Actively pull your abdominals up and in.
- Push away from the floor (rather than collapsing down) to engage your core.
- Focus on the *pulling in* of the knee rather than the extending of the leg. This will engage your abdominals more fully and protect your feet and ankles.

Intermediate Progression

Increase speed.

Advanced Progression

Keep your foot off the floor as you bring your knee in.

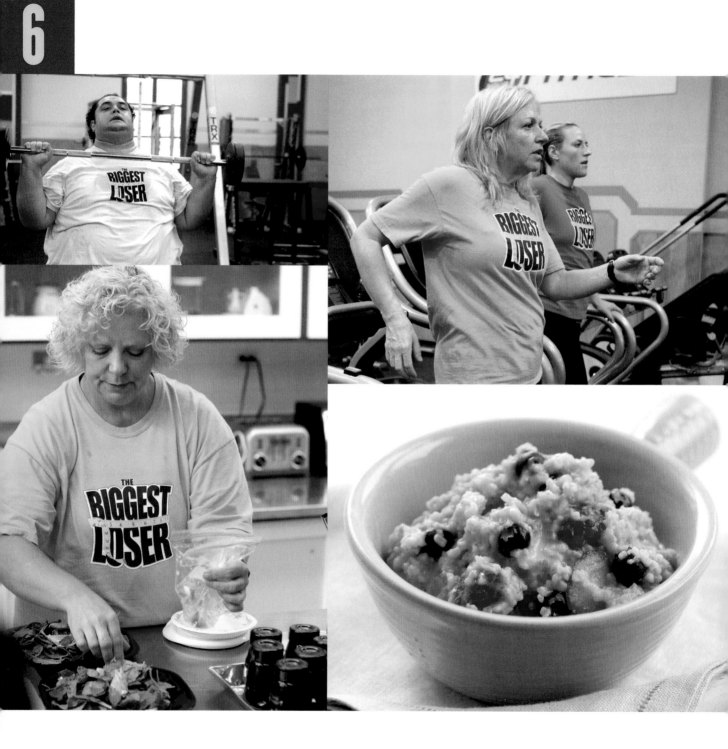

6

Week 3: Cut Your Cancer Risk

As Dr. Huizenga admits, the stakes seem to grow higher with each new crop of *Biggest Loser* contestants. Season 9 is no exception. "This is far and away the most unhealthy, catastrophic group we've had," he commented. He was referring to their high risk profile for developing obesity-related diseases. Dr. Huizenga's goal is to reverse and prevent serious diseases—such as cancer—before they have a chance to develop.

Season 9 contestant Cherita Andrews is no stranger to cancer, having fought and beaten breast cancer at the age of 38. "I decided then that death was not an option, and now at age 50 I've decided death is still no longer an option. I cannot afford to die. I want to prove to women at all ages that they can lose weight," she says.

When she and daughter Vicky were eliminated early in the competition, Cherita says she knew their weight-loss journey would continue at home. "Everybody has a story, something that life has thrown at them. Right after that devastating moment, when I realized we

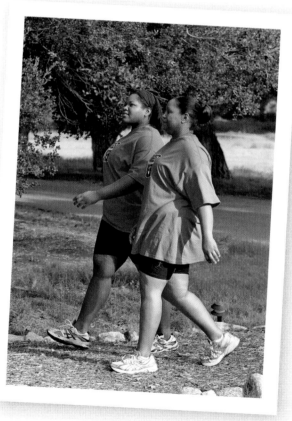

weren't going to stay on the Ranch, the next couple of days we hiked to the top of a mountain. I had never done that in my life; it was previously unfathomable to me. I realized then there is absolutely nothing that we can't do."

Quitting smoking is, of course, a no-brainer when it comes to preventing diseases like cancer. Season 9 mom Cheryl George received sobering news from Dr. Huizenga during her first week on the Ranch when he told her that although she was 51, her body's real age was 75. Half of that aging and damage had come from smoking cigarettes, he told her, and the other half was obesity and obesity-related problems. Since she was on the Ranch with her son and teammate, Daris, Dr. Huizenga drove home the point: "You're the mom. You've got to set an example."

Cheryl quit smoking cold turkey at the Ranch

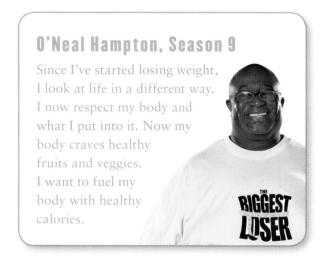

O'Neal Hampton, Season 9

Since I've started losing weight, I look at life in a different way. I now respect my body and what I put into it. Now my body craves healthy fruits and veggies. I want to fuel my body with healthy calories.

and hasn't wavered from that commitment. Recently, she said she understood that the road to health was a disciplined one, and it didn't include cigarettes. "If I can quit cigarettes," she says, "then I know anyone can do anything they put their mind to."

Season 7 winner Helen Phillips stubbed out one of her last cigarettes while having her publicity pictures taken before her season began. She knew she had gotten to the "do or die" place in her life. "I'm proud to say that I do not smoke anymore," she says today. "I stopped when I got to the Ranch, and I still had smoker's cough for about 6 weeks after that. But then I stopped coughing and started running!" Nothing has slowed Helen down since.

Coach Mo DeWalt of Season 8 admits that he still struggles with cigarettes. It's one bad habit he has yet to kick. But he has cut back on the number of cigarettes he smokes, and he says he knows that knowledge and commitment will see him through kicking his addiction, just as they did for overeating.

After heart disease, cancer is the second leading cause of death in the United States. In addition to kicking smoking to the curb, you can make other lifestyle changes to cut your cancer risk—including losing weight, eating a diet rich in cancer-fighting foods, and getting plenty of exercise. What more incentive do you need to start getting healthy today?

What Causes Cancer?

As adults, most of us know how to play well with others, follow the rules, and do our jobs. The same is true for the trillions of cells in our bodies. All cells contain "instructions" in their genes that tell them how to behave properly—how to form tissues and organs, how to replace other injured cells, and even how to die after they've become too damaged to function properly. Normally our cells follow the rules, but sometimes a rebel cell emerges and disobeys instructions. This renegade cell can cause cancer.

There are many things that can damage the genetic instructions that keep your cells operating properly. Certain chemicals, such as those found in cigarette smoke and nitrates (found in cured, processed meats), can cause this damage, as can ultraviolet rays from the sun.

Another major cause of cell damage is free radicals—oxygen molecules with one or more unpaired electrons. These molecules zip around in your body, trying to steal electrons from or donate them to other molecules, turning them into free radicals in the process. Your body creates a steady flow of these troublemakers during everyday metabolism, using at least 2 percent of the oxygen you breathe to make free radicals. The damage free radicals cause is called oxidation or oxidative stress, and it can trigger DNA mutations in cells.

Darrell Hough, Season 9

I love to walk. It allows me to get things right in my head. At home, I didn't take time for me. Now while walking, I get two great benefits: one for the body and one for the mind.

Damaged cells often die on their own or are wiped out by your immune system. But sometimes a wayward cell escapes—and then it divides, reproduces, and creates more abnormal cells at an accelerated rate. The growing collection of cancer cells—a tumor—may damage surrounding tissue. In response, your body grows blood vessels around the damaged tissue, supplying it with food and depriving other tissues and organs of nutrition. Eventually, the cancer cells may enter a blood vessel or the lymph system and spread to other parts of the body.

Different types of cancer are classified according to where they originate in the body. The chart on page 128 lists the American Cancer Society's (ACS) estimates of the leading types of new cancer diagnoses in 2009.

Leading Sites of New Cancer Cases

Men	Women
Prostate (25%)	Breast (27%)
Lung and bronchus (15%)	Lung and bronchus (14%)
Colon and rectum (10%)	Colon and rectum (10%)
Urinary bladder (7%)	Uterine corpus (6%)
Melanoma of the skin (5%)	Non-Hodgkin's lymphoma (4%)

Source: *American Cancer Society*

Risk Factors

Cancer has a reputation for striking suddenly and at random; it's true that anyone can get it, regardless of their risk profile. While those with a family history of cancer are at an elevated risk of developing the disease, the ACS estimates that only about 5 percent of cancers are strongly hereditary and that most cancers result from genetic damage occurring during one's lifetime. Perhaps for that reason, age is a primary risk factor for cancer. About 77 percent of all cancers are diagnosed in people 55 years and older.

But beyond hereditary genetics and the natural

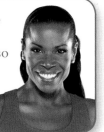

Nicole Brewer, Season 7

My quality of life has changed so much. At 39, I'm proud of what I've accomplished. I just ran my first marathon!

Shay Sorrells, Season 8

I'm a convert to Spinning classes. The first one may be rough, but after you get through it, you feel so great. After an hour of Spinning and sweating tons, my legs are a little like Jell-O, but I feel amazing. That's an exercise I'm going to keep doing the rest of my life.

process of aging, you have the power to eliminate or change many cancer risk factors, including:

- **Smoking.** About 30 percent of cancers are caused by exposure to cigarette smoke and other forms of tobacco. By not using tobacco—and avoiding other people's smoke—you improve your odds of remaining cancer free.
- **Poor diet.** Another 15 percent of cancers are linked to dietary factors: problems like too many calories, too much fat, too many harmful chemicals in certain foods, too few vegetables, and too little fiber.
- **Hormones.** Another 30 percent or so, including breast and endometrial cancers, are linked to the influence of hormones. Your food choices may help lower your risk of these cancers, too.

Pop Quiz: Nutrition

In Season 8, the contestants participated in a pop quiz challenge to test their nutrition smarts. Answer the questions below and see how you score!

1. Name three different ways to cook without using oil.

2. How many calories are in a typical chain restaurant chicken Caesar salad?

   A. 540 calories
   B. 840 calories
   C. 1,010 calories

3. When you substitute sliced zucchini for pasta, how many calories do you eliminate from one serving?

   A. 110 calories
   B. 248 calories
   C. 343 calories

4. How many calories would you consume if you drank one 16-ounce soda with three refills?

   A. 685 calories
   B. 747 calories
   C. 789 calories

5. Which of these desserts has fewer than 150 calories?

   A. A cup of fresh raspberries with ½ ounce melted dark chocolate dipping sauce

   B. A parfait of 1 cup blueberries with ½ cup low-fat yogurt and 1 tablespoon slivered almonds

   C. A cup of vanilla ice cream

6. Name two reasons why it's important to add a protein to any snack.

Answers: 1. Bake, poach, or steam. 2. **A.** 3. **B.** 4. **B.** 5. **A.** 6. To help you feel fuller and to help repair muscles.

According to the American Cancer Society (ACS), the second-best way to cut your cancer risk (after quitting smoking) is to "achieve and maintain a healthy weight, to be physically active on a regular basis, and to make healthy food choices." Eating right, exercising, and not smoking won't guarantee that you will remain cancer free, but making these changes in your lifestyle will greatly reduce your risk.

The Weight-Loss Connection

Being overweight and leading a sedentary lifestyle are linked to many kinds of cancers, including those of the colon, kidney, and breast. According to the ACS, about one-third of the 562,340 cancer deaths expected to occur in 2009 will be related to overweight or obesity, physical inactivity, and poor nutrition—and thus may have been preventable.

Calorie restriction might help prevent cancer by reducing inflammation, promoting DNA repair, and encouraging cells to die as programmed (a process called apoptosis). Following your calorie budget on *The Biggest Loser* eating plan will help you maintain a healthy weight or shed unnecessary pounds.

Getting 30 minutes of exercise daily will help, too. A physically active lifestyle has been linked to a lower risk of many cancers, including colon cancer in women.

The Antioxidant Power of Fruits and Vegetables

You can strengthen your body's protection against damage from free radicals by eating a diet rich in antioxidants.

Your body creates powerful antioxidant enzymes and bolsters its defenses with nutrients from your food choices. Dietary antioxidants include vitamins A, C, and E; minerals that support your body's antioxidant enzymes; and certain plant chemicals called phytochemicals.

A new measurement unit called the ORAC (oxygen radical absorbance capacity) score measures the antioxidant levels in foods. The chart on the opposite page provides a listing of foods with the highest ORAC scores.

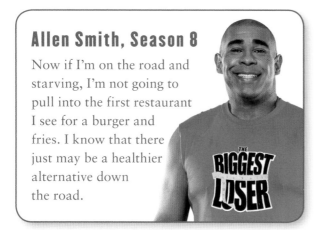

Allen Smith, Season 8

Now if I'm on the road and starving, I'm not going to pull into the first restaurant I see for a burger and fries. I know that there just may be a healthier alternative down the road.

Antioxidant Food Sources

Food	Serving size	ORAC
Sorghum flour	¼ c	9,378
Beans, mature small red, dry	¼ c	6,864
Blueberries, lowbush (wild)	½ c	6,314
Blackstrap molasses	1 Tbsp	5,366
Red wine	6 oz	4,585
Natural cocoa powder	1 Tbsp	4,100
Artichoke hearts, cooked	½ c	3,952
Dried plums	¼ c	3,646
Cloves, ground	½ tsp	3,144
Green tea, brewed	1 c	2,951
Coffee, brewed	1 c	2,860
Pecans	2 Tbsp	2,548
Ginger, fresh, chopped	2 Tbsp	1,781
Tarragon, fresh	1 Tbsp	933
Extra-virgin olive oil	2 Tbsp	303

To boost your antioxidant power:

- **"Paint your plate" with colorful fruits and vegetables.** The phytochemicals found in fruits and vegetables can help prevent cancer in many different ways, including but not limited to their antioxidant power. In one study, men and women had up to a 15 percent increase in the antioxidant power of their blood after increasing their daily fruit and vegetable intake, compared with what they consumed before the study. Season 8 contestant Abby Rike says she's already noticing the positive changes in her body that have resulted from eating more nutritious foods. "Small, simple changes in your diet will yield big results. I realize that the garbage I was putting into my body before did nothing to enhance the quality of my life. I now incorporate fresh fruit and vegetables. They truly make you start feeling better from the inside out." To boost your fruit and vegetable intake:

- Add fresh or dried fruits like chopped apples, raisins, prunes, kiwifruit, or orange sections to green leafy salads.
- Make stir-fries or casseroles with lots of vegetables.
- Think fruit for dessert. Frozen berries make an ideal base for sorbet, while poached apples or pears are perfect warm treats. For another delicious fruit dessert, try the Apple Treat recipe on page 143.

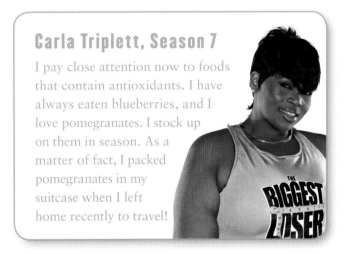

Carla Triplett, Season 7

I pay close attention now to foods that contain antioxidants. I have always eaten blueberries, and I love pomegranates. I stock up on them in season. As a matter of fact, I packed pomegranates in my suitcase when I left home recently to travel!

- **Consume antioxidant fuel throughout the day.** About 85 percent of the antioxidants in fruits and vegetables are water soluble—meaning that 5 hours after you eat a piece of produce, most of its antioxidant benefits have left your system. That's why you should make sure you have a good source of antioxidants every few hours throughout the day. Choose fresh fruits and veggies for on-the-go snacks. Season 9 contestant Sam Poueu says he's found an easy way to get in his veggies every day: He makes quick veggie stir-fries. "I was never a big fan of vegetables before, but at the Ranch you realize how big a role they play in a healthy diet," he adds.

  See the chart at left for a list of cancer-fighting foods you can easily incorporate into your diet.

- **Skip the pills.** Antioxidants found in food are much more effective and safer (not to mention cheaper) than those found in over-the-counter supplements. When it comes to antioxidants, Mother Nature knows best!

Anti-Cancer Powerfoods

Choose these antioxidant-rich fruits and vegetables for cancer prevention:

- Apples
- Blueberries
- Broccoli
- Brussels sprouts
- Cabbage
- Carrots
- Cranberries
- Grapefruit
- Grapes
- Green and black tea
- Kale
- Mustard greens
- Onions
- Spinach
- Strawberries
- Sweet potatoes
- Tomatoes

Meat in Moderation

Red meat has been linked to an increased risk of colon cancer—the second-deadliest cancer, after lung cancer. Processed or cured meats pose an additional risk: They contain preservatives called nitrites and nitrates, which can be converted in your stomach to substances called nitrosamines—which are linked to an increased risk of cancer of the stomach and some other organs.

When it comes to protein, choose lean poultry, fish, or red meat as the side dish to vegetables, rather than vice versa. Season 6 contestant Vicky Vilcan says she rarely eats red meat anymore and

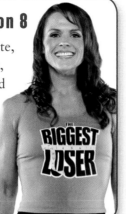

Tracey Yukich, Season 8

When you prepare your plate, reserve one-half for veggies, one-quarter for protein, and one-quarter for complex carbs like whole grains. That way, you can quickly eyeball if you're eating the right balance of nutrients.

chooses healthier proteins. "I now eat leaner cuts of meat like chicken, turkey, and fish. They all contain less saturated fat than beef does. I can eat more chicken, turkey, and fish than I can red meats and I still feel satisfied."

To make healthy meat choices:

- **Stick with fresh, unprocessed meat.** Avoid pickled, salted, or cured meats, including bacon, hot dogs, store-bought jerky, and processed deli meats. If you do have an occasional hankering for bacon, choose nitrate-free turkey bacon, available in most health food stores. Season 8 winner Danny Cahill says he's a convert to turkey bacon. "It's one of the most amazing foods I discovered at the Ranch. It's so satisfying. You can whip up a quick meal with a whole wheat tortilla, turkey bacon, and fresh chopped veggies and tomato. You're ready to go in 5 minutes."

- **Don't overcook.** Cooking meats at high temperatures causes formation of heterocyclic amines (HCAs) and polycyclic aromatic hydrocarbons (PAHs). HCAs are formed in muscle meats at high temperatures. PAHs result from fat dripping onto hot coals during grilling or barbecuing, which creates smoke that then collects on the meat. Both of these chemicals are suspected to be carcinogenic in humans. To avoid them:
  - Stick with cooking methods that don't char your food. Roasting or baking can add a layer of rich flavor without charring.
  - When you do use a grill, drain and blot away any excess oil if marinating the meat.
  - Place your food on foil to prevent fat from dripping on the coals, and cut off any portion of food that gets blackened.

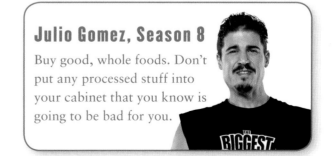

Julio Gomez, Season 8

Buy good, whole foods. Don't put any processed stuff into your cabinet that you know is going to be bad for you.

Week 3 Menu Plan

MONDAY — 1,460 calories

Breakfast

Berry-licious Oatmeal (page 141)

3 slices turkey bacon

1 hard-boiled egg

1 cup fat-free milk

Green tea or coffee

Snack

½ tuna salad sandwich on whole grain bread

Lunch

2 cups low-fat minestrone

¾ cup fat-free vanilla yogurt with ⅓ cup raspberries

Iced tea

Snack

Bye-Bye Blues Smoothie (page 150)

Dinner

5 ounces tilapia, baked, with lemon wedge

8 medium spears asparagus, steamed or grilled

2 Roma tomatoes roasted with 1 teaspoon olive oil, ½ teaspoon minced garlic, and 1 tablespoon chopped basil

1 cup fat-free milk

Green tea or coffee

TUESDAY — 1,540 calories

Breakfast

2 whole grain toaster waffles

1 poached egg

2 slices Canadian bacon

½ large pink grapefruit

1 cup fat-free milk

Green tea or coffee

Snack

1 large wedge cantaloupe (⅛ of large melon)

2 ounces roast turkey

Lunch

1 serving **White Chicken Chili** (page 179)

2 cups mixed greens with 1 tablespoon low-fat balsamic dressing

1 cup red or green grapes

Iced green or black tea

Snack

2 medium tangerines and ½ ounce walnuts

Dinner

5 ounces calamari sautéed with 1 teaspoon olive oil, 1 cup fire-roasted tomatoes, 1 teaspoon minced garlic, and 1 teaspoon fresh thyme

3 cups baby spinach, steamed

Apple Treat (page 143)

1 cup fat-free milk

Green tea

WEDNESDAY   1,550 calories

Breakfast

Yogurt parfait: 1 cup plain, fat-free Greek-style yogurt; ½ teaspoon vanilla extract; 1 cup berries (blueberries, strawberries, raspberries, or combination); and ⅓ cup low-fat granola

1 large orange

Green tea or coffee

Snack

1 cup steamed edamame

Lunch

1 cup whole grain pasta with ½ cup low-fat marinara sauce and 1 grilled low-fat turkey Italian sausage

2 cups baby spinach with 1 tablespoon low-fat Caesar dressing and 1 teaspoon grated Parmesan cheese

1 cup fat-free milk

Snack

½ chicken and cheese quesadilla made with 1 corn tortilla; 1 slice low-fat mozzarella or provolone cheese; and 1 ounce roasted chicken breast, shredded

Dinner

1 serving **Pork Tenderloin with Warm Asian Slaw** (page 147)

Sliced tomatoes drizzled with 1 teaspoon low-sodium soy sauce, 1 teaspoon rice wine vinegar, and 1 teaspoon chopped cilantro

1 pear

Green tea

THURSDAY   1,525 calories

Breakfast

3 egg whites (½ cup) scrambled with 1 teaspoon olive oil, 1 teaspoon chopped basil, 1 teaspoon grated Parmesan cheese, and ½ cup cherry tomatoes

1 slice whole grain toast

1 cup fat-free milk

½ cup fresh blueberries

Decaf iced tea with lemon

Snack

½ cup fat-free vanilla yogurt (or frozen yogurt) sprinkled with 2 tablespoons sliced strawberries

Lunch

Chicken and rice salad: 4 ounces grilled chicken breast, chopped; ¾ cup cooked brown rice; and 1 cup diced grilled vegetables (2 tablespoons onion, ¼ cup zucchini, ½ cup bell pepper)

1 teaspoon chopped cilantro with 1 tablespoon low-fat vinaigrette and 1 tablespoon shredded low-fat Cheddar cheese

Ice water with lime

Snack

2 tablespoons hummus and ½ cup jicama slices

Dinner

4-ounce wild salmon fillet, grilled

1 cup wild rice

1 cup wilted baby spinach with 1 teaspoon olive oil, 1 teaspoon balsamic vinegar, and 1 teaspoon grated Parmesan cheese

½ cup fresh berries with ½ cup orange sorbet and 1 teaspoon chopped almonds

FRIDAY   1,510 calories

Breakfast

½ cup fresh diced melon

½ cup old-fashioned oatmeal (cooked in 1 cup water with 1 tablespoon ground flaxseed) sprinkled with ground cinnamon and 1 tablespoon chopped pecans

½ cup fat-free vanilla yogurt

Mint tea

Snack

1 fresh pear, sliced and topped with ½ cup fat-free ricotta cheese and 1 teaspoon honey

Lunch

Mediterranean turkey pita sandwich: 4½ ounces thinly sliced lean turkey breast, ½ roasted red bell pepper, 2 pieces romaine lettuce, and **Avocado Green Goddess Dip or Dressing** (page 148) in 1 whole wheat pita (4" diameter)

Sparkling water with orange slice

Snack

1 stick fat-free mozzarella string cheese

1 medium orange

Dinner

5 ounces flank steak grilled with 2 Roma tomatoes

Large tossed salad: 2 cups mixed greens, ¼ cup sliced cucumbers, ¼ cup sliced mushrooms, and 2 tablespoons light Caesar dressing

¾ cup whole wheat couscous

1 cup fat-free milk

SATURDAY   1,545 calories

Breakfast

Breakfast burrito: 4 egg whites (⅔ cup) scrambled with 1 teaspoon olive oil, ¼ cup fat-free refried black beans, 2 tablespoons salsa, 2 tablespoons grated low-fat pepper Jack cheese, and 1 teaspoon cilantro on 1 medium whole wheat tortilla

1 cup mixed diced melon

Iced tea

Snack

1 large apple, sliced, with 1 tablespoon almond butter or peanut butter

Lunch

4-ounce chicken breast, grilled

½ cup cooked lentils heated with 1 tablespoon low-sugar barbecue sauce and 1 teaspoon chopped cilantro

Spinach salad: 1 cup baby spinach leaves, ¼ cup halved cherry tomatoes, 1 tablespoon light Russian vinaigrette, and 2 teaspoons grated Parmesan cheese

1 cup fat-free milk

Snack

1 stick low-fat mozzarella string cheese

1 cup red grapes

Dinner

4 ounces pork tenderloin stir-fried with 1 cup broccoli, 1 teaspoon garlic, and 1 teaspoon low-sodium soy sauce

½ cup cooked brown rice or bulgur wheat

5 medium tomato slices with 1 teaspoon balsamic vinegar and 1 teaspoon chopped fresh basil

Herbal tea

Banana Fudge Smoothie (page 150)

SUNDAY   1,520 calories

Breakfast

1 egg and 2 large egg whites scrambled with ¼ cup shredded low-fat pepper Jack cheese and 1 teaspoon chopped cilantro

1 wedge honeydew melon

1 slice whole grain bread, toasted

1 cup fat-free milk

Snack

1 medium apple and ½ ounce raw almonds

Lunch

Roast beef wrap: 4 ounces thinly sliced lean roast beef (or chicken, turkey, or pork), ¼ cup shredded lettuce, 3 medium tomato slices, 1 teaspoon horseradish, and 1 teaspoon Dijon mustard in 1 whole wheat tortilla (6" diameter)

½ cup jicama sticks

½ cup cooked pinto beans or lentils with 1 teaspoon chopped basil and 1 tablespoon light Caesar vinaigrette

Iced decaf coffee

Snack

8 baked corn tortilla chips with 2 tablespoons guacamole and 2 tablespoons salsa

Dinner

4-ounce salmon or halibut fillet, grilled

½ cup sliced mushrooms sautéed with 1 teaspoon olive oil, ¼ cup chopped yellow onion, and ¼ cup sliced bell pepper

1 cup arugula salad with ½ cup halved cherry tomatoes and 1 tablespoon low-fat miso dressing

½ cup warm unsweetened applesauce with ¼ cup fat-free vanilla yogurt, dash of ground cinnamon, and 1 tablespoon chopped pecans

Green or mint tea

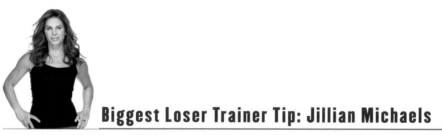

Biggest Loser Trainer Tip: Jillian Michaels

If you're a fan of mashed potatoes, you can still have them without the guilt. But substitute cauliflower for those starchy potatoes. The texture and the taste are similar, and you're getting your daily vegetables in. Cauliflower is high in dietary fiber, potassium, vitamin B$_6$, and vitamin C. And it has no saturated fat. And zero cholesterol.

STEEL-CUT OATS

Many people miss out on the fabulous flavor and texture of steel-cut oats because this grain requires more cooking time than old-fashioned or instant oats, and preparing it means standing over the stove the whole time. Here's a quick cooking tip that will allow you to squeeze in a workout (or at least a few situps) while your breakfast is almost making itself!

4 cups Almond Breeze unsweetened vanilla almond milk or 4 cups water

1 cup steel-cut oats

Pinch of salt

In a 2-quart saucepan, bring the almond milk or water to a low boil. Add the oats and salt, reduce the heat, and simmer for a few minutes. Cover the pan and remove from the heat. Cool to room temperature (about 1 hour). Store in the refrigerator or freezer and reheat as needed.

Note: Cooking the oats in water instead of almond milk will reduce the calories to 140 per serving.

Makes 4 (1-cup) servings

Per serving: 180 calories, 7 g protein, 29 g carbohydrates (0 g sugars), 6 g fat (< 1 g saturated), 0 mg cholesterol, 5 g fiber, 180 mg sodium

Rebecca Meyer, Season 8

Exercise is paramount for weight loss. You need to push yourself to the point where you almost feel like you can't go anymore. Living healthy has really changed my energy level. And the food I'm eating is not slowing me down anymore because it's not full of fat!

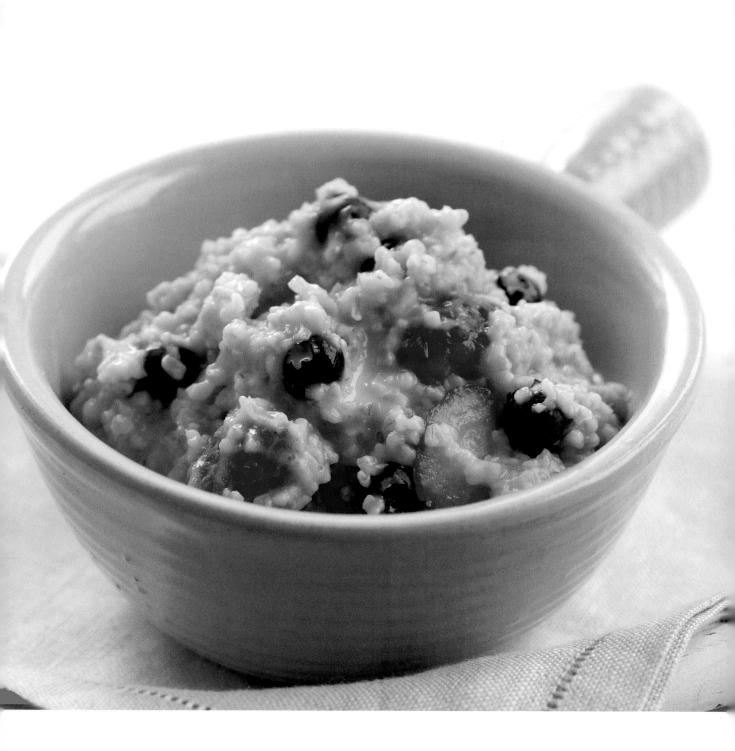

BERRY-LICIOUS OATMEAL

Season 8's Shay Sorrells says, "I'm really busy, so I always buy precooked steel-cut oats, which makes this an easy breakfast recipe." (See the "Steel-Cut Oats" recipe on page 139 to cook oats in advance.) You can use any combination of fresh or frozen (and thawed) berries for this delicious, fruit-packed start to your day.

1 cup cooked steel-cut oats

2 tablespoons fresh or frozen blueberries

2 tablespoons fresh or frozen raspberries

½ cup sliced strawberries

1 teaspoon vanilla extract

¼ cup Almond Breeze unsweetened vanilla almond milk

1 packet Truvia or other natural sweetener

Combine the oats, berries, vanilla, almond milk, and sweetener in a cereal bowl and stir well. Microwave for 1 to 2 minutes and serve.

Makes 1 serving

Per serving: 220 calories, 7 g protein, 39 g carbohydrates (8 g sugars), 4 g fat (0 g saturated), 0 mg cholesterol, 7 g fiber, 50 mg sodium

Julie Hadden, Season 4 Finalist

I've learned that I'm stronger than I ever thought I could possibly be, that I am worthy to live the life I dreamed of. I didn't believe that before.

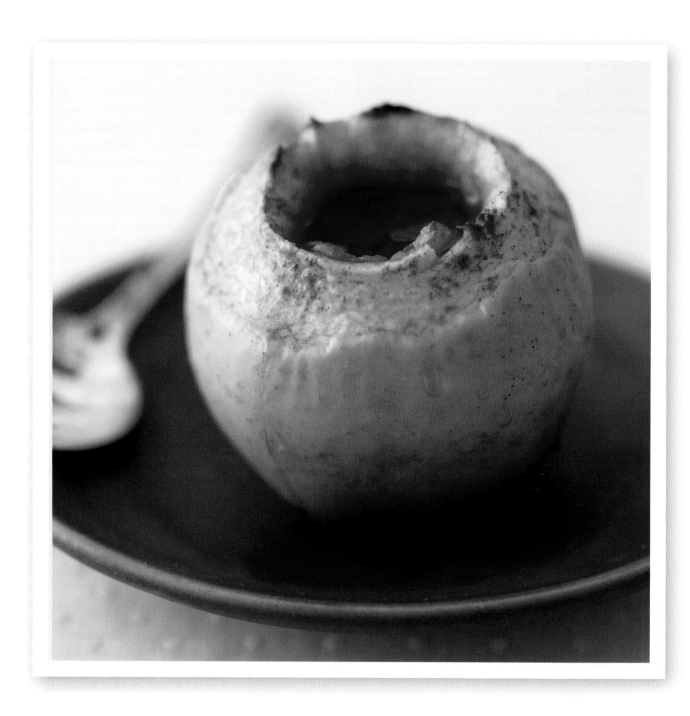

APPLE TREAT

This easy dessert contains all the natural goodness of an apple, including plenty of fiber. It is especially delicious on a cool autumn evening, when apples are at their peak of freshness.

1 large (3¼") Golden Delicious apple

1 teaspoon ground cinnamon

2 teaspoons Truvia or other natural sweetener

Preheat the oven to 375°F. Using a sharp paring knife, core the apple ¾ of the way through, leaving a ½" seal at the bottom. Trim the skin around the top of the apple. Place the apple in an ungreased baking dish. Combine the cinnamon and sweetener and pour most of the mixture into the center of the apple; sprinkle the rest on top of the apple and in the bottom of the baking dish. Pour water ¼" deep in the baking dish.

Bake uncovered for 30 to 40 minutes, until the apple is tender. Spoon the mixture in the baking dish over the apple while it is baking.

Makes 1 serving

Per serving: **120 calories, 1 g protein, 32 g carbohydrates (22 g sugars), 0 g fat (0 g saturated), 0 mg cholesterol, 6 g fiber, 0 mg sodium**

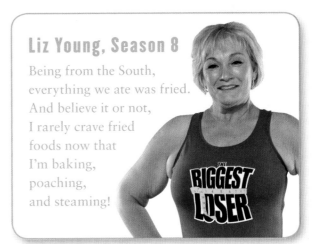

Liz Young, Season 8

Being from the South, everything we ate was fried. And believe it or not, I rarely crave fried foods now that I'm baking, poaching, and steaming!

AVOCADO AND APPLE CHICKEN SALAD

This recipe was inspired by my friend Chef Roberto Santibañez. I love the richness of avocado combined with the sweet crispness of apples in this delicious, filling salad. It's perfect for lunch.

- 2 cups (about 12 ounces) cooked chicken or turkey breast, cut in 1" pieces
- 1 cup diced sweet red apple
- ½ cup thinly sliced celery
- ¼ cup lightly toasted pecans, coarsely chopped
- ½ cup roughly chopped flat-leaf (Italian) parsley
- ¼ cup chopped red onion
- 1½ tablespoons chopped mint (about 10 leaves)
- 1½ tablespoons chopped jalapeño pepper (optional)
- ½ teaspoon salt
- 2 tablespoons lemon juice
- 1 teaspoon olive oil
- 1 fully ripened avocado, halved, pitted, peeled, and diced
- 4 cups mixed baby salad greens

In a large bowl, combine the chicken, apple, celery, pecans, parsley, onion, mint, jalapeño pepper (if desired), salt, lemon juice, and oil; stir. Add the avocado; toss gently until all the ingredients are combined, leaving some diced avocado visible while mashing some. Serve over the mixed greens.

Makes 4 servings

Per serving: 200 calories, 17 g protein, 14 g carbohydrates (5 g sugars), 12 g fat (1 g saturated), 30 mg cholesterol, 4 g fiber, 340 mg sodium

Koli Palu, Season 9

Losing weight creates such a feeling of pride. I am so proud of what I'm accomplishing. In the past, I was always worried about my future, knowing how unhealthy I was. Now that I've taken control of my health and taken ownership, my worries are disappearing.

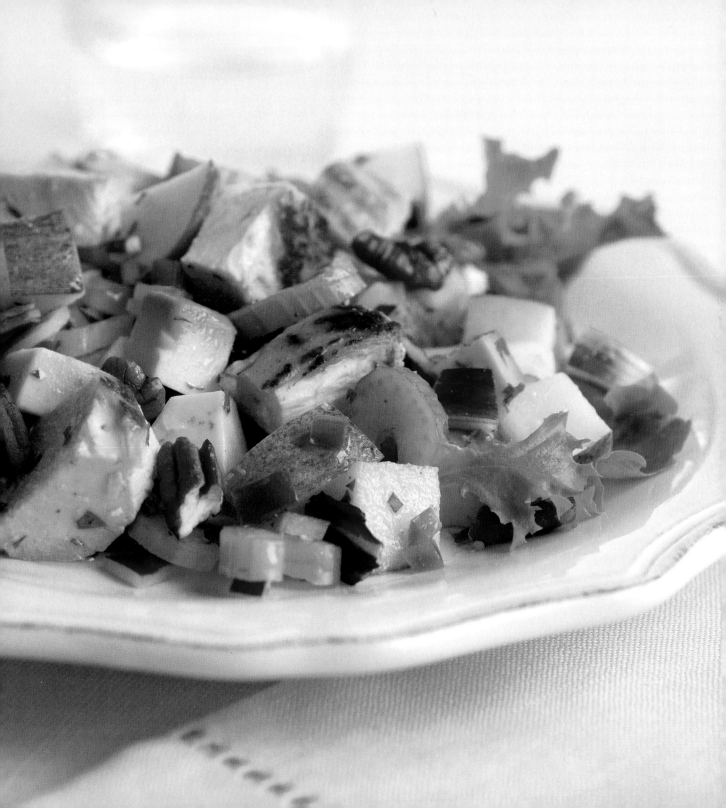

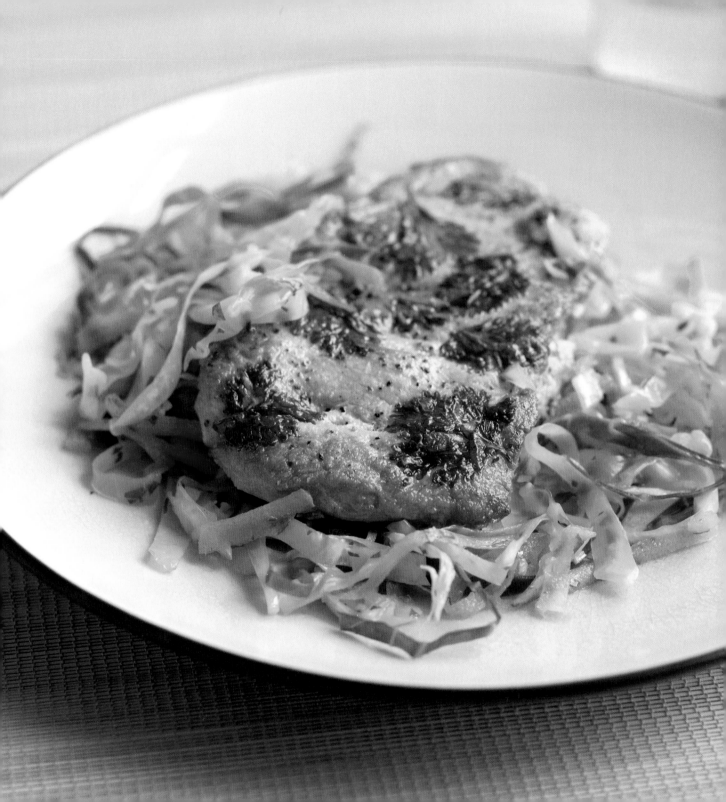

PORK TENDERLOIN WITH WARM ASIAN SLAW

Cilantro-crusted pork tenderloin is full of flavor. Paired with a zesty Asian slaw, this dish is a delicious twist on the same old pork tenderloin.

Slaw

- 2 teaspoons olive oil
- 1 medium yellow onion, finely chopped
- 1 tablespoon minced garlic
- 1 tablespoon chopped, peeled fresh ginger
- 3 cups finely shredded green cabbage
- ½ cup grated carrot
- 1 tablespoon low-sodium soy sauce
- ⅓ cup chopped cilantro, without stems
  Salt to taste

Pork

- 4 (4-ounce) pieces lean pork tenderloin
- ¼ teaspoon salt
- ⅛ teaspoon ground black pepper
- 1½ tablespoons chopped cilantro + cilantro sprigs for garnish
- 1 teaspoon olive oil

To make the slaw: In a large skillet, heat 2 teaspoons olive oil over medium-high heat. Add the onion and cook for about 2 minutes, until softened but not colored. Add the garlic and ginger and cook for 1 minute longer. Add the cabbage and stir-fry for about 2 minutes longer.

Remove the pan from the heat. Add the carrot, soy sauce, and ⅓ cup chopped cilantro. Stir until combined. Season with salt, if desired. There should be about 2 cups of slaw. Keep the slaw warm.

To make the pork: Place the pork tenderloin between 2 sheets of heavy-duty plastic wrap. With a meat mallet or rolling pin, pound each piece to an even ¼" thickness. Sprinkle with the salt and pepper. Dredge the pork in the chopped cilantro, pressing to make the leaves stick.

In a large nonstick skillet, heat the oil over medium-high heat. Add the pork to the pan and cook for 2 to 3 minutes per side, until opaque throughout and tender.

To serve: Place the pork on individual serving plates and top each piece with ¼ of the Asian Slaw. Garnish with a sprig of cilantro, if desired.

Makes 4 servings

> **Per serving:** 200 calories, 2 g protein, 8 g carbohydrates (4 g sugars), 7 g fat (2 g saturated), 75 mg cholesterol, 2 g fiber, 210 mg sodium

AVOCADO GREEN GODDESS DIP OR DRESSING

When I was trying to create a dip that didn't contain mayonnaise or sour cream, I decided to replace those condiments' unhealthy fats with the creamy richness (and healthy fats!) of avocado. This delicious dip makes a great snack with fresh cut veggies, and it can also be used as a salad dressing. To make the dressing, add a little extra buttermilk to thin the mixture.

1½ cups plain, fat-free Greek-style yogurt

½ cup low-fat buttermilk

½ medium ripe avocado, diced

1 tablespoon chopped basil

1 tablespoon chopped cilantro

1 teaspoon Worcestershire sauce

1 teaspoon dried dill

1 teaspoon ground mustard

1 teaspoon garlic powder

1 teaspoon onion powder

½ teaspoon ground black pepper

½ to 1 teaspoon salt (optional)

Combine the yogurt, buttermilk, avocado, basil, cilantro, Worcestershire sauce, dill, mustard, garlic powder, onion powder, black pepper, and salt (if desired) in a food processor or blender. Process or blend until smooth. Store in the refrigerator. The dressing keeps about 3 days.

Makes 8 (¼-cup) servings, or 2 cups

Per serving: 50 calories, 5 g protein, 3 g carbohydrates (2 g sugars), 2 g fat (0 g saturated), 0 mg cholesterol, 1 g fiber, 30 mg sodium

Stephanie Anderson, Season 9

I love Greek yogurt—add some Truvia and berries for a complete meal full of protein and low in calories!

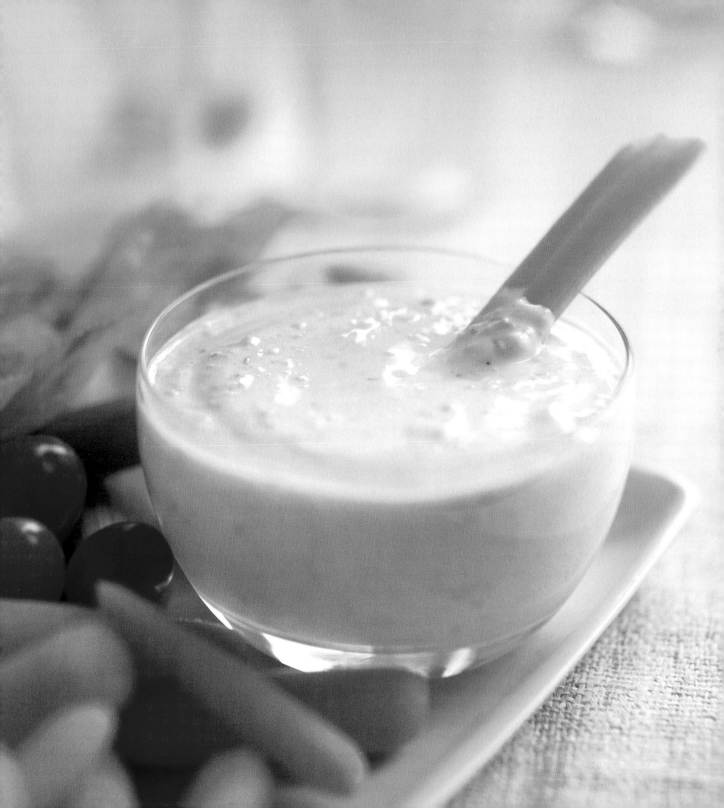

BYE-BYE BLUES SMOOTHIE

Named for its vibrant color, this smoothie can be enjoyed year-round, since you can use fresh or frozen fruit. This is Season 5 winner Ali Vincent's all-time favorite!

1 scoop (4 tablespoons) *The Biggest Loser* blueberry protein powder

½ cup fat-free milk

½ cup fresh or frozen blueberries

½ cup fresh or frozen blackberries

Combine the protein powder, milk, blueberries, and blackberries in a blender or food processor. Blend or process until smooth. Pour into a glass and serve immediately.

Makes 1 smoothie

Per serving: 120 calories, 8 g protein, 26 g carbohydrates (12 g sugars), 2 g fat (0 g saturated), 0 mg cholesterol, 11 g fiber, 60 mg sodium

BANANA FUDGE SMOOTHIE

This fudgy, creamy treat is great for a midday pick-me-up. It's loaded with protein and fiber.

¾ cups very cold unsweetened vanilla almond milk

¼ cup plain, fat-free Greek-style yogurt

1 ripe medium banana, frozen and cut into 1" chunks

1 scoop (4 tablespoons) *The Biggest Loser* chocolate protein powder

1 tablespoon unsweetened natural cocoa powder

½ teaspoon vanilla extract

1 packet natural sweetener

Combine the all ingredients in a blender or food processor. Blend or process until smooth. Pour the smoothie into a glass and serve immediately.

Makes 1 (1½-cup) serving

Per serving: 240 calories, 14 g protein, 43 g carbohydrates (24 g sugars), 4 g fat (0 g saturated), 0 mg cholesterol, 13 g fiber, 210 mg sodium

Shay Sorrells, Season 8

After my time at the Ranch, I drank almond milk. I love making fruit smoothies with frozen blueberries and almond milk.

Week 3 Exercises

The fitness goals for the first 2 weeks of the plan focused on body-weight training to develop muscle tone, joint mobility, and flexibility and on aerobic training for heart health and overall fitness. The benefits of strength training include:

- increased bone density
- increased lean body mass (more muscle, less fat!)
- heightened metabolism
- a more functional and balanced body

Recent studies have shown that strength/resistance training can boost cancer prevention and recovery. Incorporating the types of exercises detailed in this chapter into your fitness program is extremely beneficial for your overall health.

The American Sports Medicine Institute states that the goal of strength training is to gradually and progressively overload the musculoskeletal system so that it becomes stronger. For our workout this week, we are going to perform compound strength exercises (upper- and lower-body moves performed at the same time) that are functional (they improve activities of daily life and sports performance) and involve more core stabilization (they actively engage the abdominal and back muscles to support the spine).

Focus: Strength/Resistance Training

Workout Guidelines

- All you need are sets of dumbbells that will fatigue your muscles in the allotted number of repetitions. As you progress and get stronger, increase the weight or resistance.
- Warm up for 5 minutes by marching in place or walking.
- Perform 10 to 15 repetitions for (one set) of each exercise. Over the course of Week 3, gradually increase to three sets.
- Begin with the most basic variation. As you get stronger, work up to the intermediate and advanced progressions.
- Follow this workout with a gentle stretch for your legs, back, and chest as well as your biceps, triceps, and shoulders.
- For a well-rounded program, try this workout for 2 or 3 days a week in addition to cardio training 3 or 4 days a week. Alternate cardio and strength days.
- If you are recovering from cancer or surgery, consult your doctor for modifications, if necessary. Some breast cancer survivors experience lymphedema (blockage or interruption of the lymphatic system) and may need to reduce or cease resistance training until symptoms disappear.

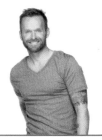

Biggest Loser Trainer Tip: Bob Harper

Keep exercise fun! Athletic leagues across the country sponsor adult softball, soccer, football, and even kickball teams. This is a great way to go if you prefer some structure, competition, and social interaction with your exercise. Find something that interests you and you'll be far more likely to stick with it.

LUNGE WITH SINGLE-ARM ROW

Begin in a staggered stance with your left leg forward and your right leg back, heel off the floor; hold a dumbbell in your right hand, with your palm facing in. Bend your left knee and hinge slightly forward at the hips, placing your left hand on your left thigh. Keeping your spine neutral and your abdominals engaged, bend both knees deeper, reaching toward the floor with the dumbbell and your right knee. As you pull the dumbbell up toward your hip, squeeze the muscles in your upper back and straighten both legs. Hold for a moment, then bend your knees and lower the dumbbell back down toward the floor. Do 10 to 15 repetitions, then switch sides (right leg forward and dumbbell in left hand) and repeat.

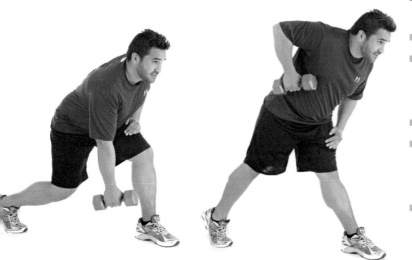

Tips

- Avoid rounding your back.
- Control the movement and don't allow your elbow to lock when you lower the dumbbell.
- Keep your navel pulled in at all times.
- In the lunge, keep your front shin perpendicular to the floor, so that your knee is directly over your ankle.
- Do not let your front knee move past your toes.

Intermediate Progression

Stretch your free arm out to the side to further involve your core.

Advanced Progression

Lift your back leg up when you raise the dumbbell, to challenge your balance.

SQUAT WITH OVERHEAD PRESS

Stand with your feet shoulder-width apart, toes pointing forward; hold a medium-to-heavy dumbbell in each hand. Bend your elbows and bring the dumbbells to your shoulders. Keep your chest lifted and your abdominals engaged. Send your hips back and bend your knees as if you were sitting in a chair, until your thighs are parallel to the floor. Push into your heels to return to standing. As you stand, press the dumbbells upward until your arms are extended overhead. Lower the weights to your shoulders as you sit back in the squat. Keep your spine neutral and your chest lifted the entire time, concentrating on coordinating the lower- and upper-body movements. Do 10 to 15 repetitions.

Tips

- Maintain your natural lower-back arch; avoid rounding your back.
- Keep your focus forward.
- As you press your arms overhead, pull your navel to your spine and don't let your back arch.

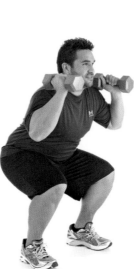
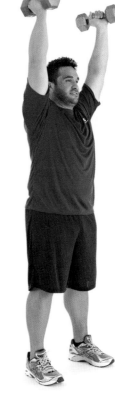

Intermediate Progression

Step out from side to side on the squat.

Advanced Progression

Lift one knee as you stand to challenge your balance.

HIP HINGE WITH TRICEPS EXTENSION

Stand with your feet shoulder-width apart, toes pointing forward; hold a light-to-medium dumbbell in each hand. Bend your elbows and bring your hands to your hips, squeezing your shoulder blades together. Keeping your knees slightly bent, bend (hinge) forward at the hips, keeping your spine neutral. Slowly extend your elbows to straighten your arms in a backward arc, squeezing your triceps (the muscles in the back of the arm). Engage your glutes (buttocks) and abdominals to lift your torso and return to standing upright as you bend your elbows to return to the starting position. Do 10 to 15 repetitions.

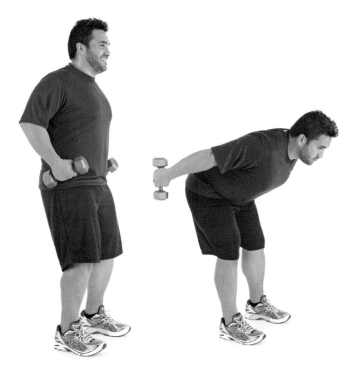

Tips

- Maintain a neutral spine and pull your shoulder blades together throughout the entire exercise. Do not allow your back to round.
- Bend only at the hips, not the spine.
- If your hamstrings are tight and your back begins to round, bend your knees a bit more to release the tension.
- Reach your knuckles to the back during the triceps extension and pull your shoulders away from your ears.

Intermediate Progression

Lift one leg back as you hinge to challenge your balance. (Alternate legs).

Advanced Progression

Hold your position in the hinge as you extend your elbows one at a time to challenge your balance and core.

PLIÉ WITH BICEPS CURL

Stand with your feet wider than your hips (2 to 3 feet apart), with your legs rotated out from the hips so that your toes point out to the sides (think 2 and 10 o'clock). Hold a medium-to-heavy dumbbell in each hand, and place your hands in front of your thighs. Bend your knees and lower your hips and torso toward the floor, keeping your back neutral and chest lifted. Make sure your knees are aligned over your feet and that they do not go past your toes. Press into the floor and return to standing while you curl the dumbbells to your shoulders. Lower the weights toward your thighs as you bend your knees to go into the next repetition. Do 10 to 15 repetitions.

Tips

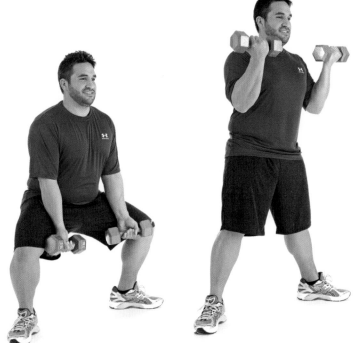

- Don't allow your body to shift forward or backward as you bend your knees.
- Imagine lengthening your spine as you lower yourself.
- Rotate from the hips, not the knees or ankles.
- Don't let your chest cave in or your shoulders roll forward when you lower the dumbbells to your thighs during the plié.

Intermediate Progression
Step out from side to side on the plié.

Advanced Progression
Lift one leg out to the side as you stand to challenge your balance.

CHEST PRESS WITH LEG PRESS

Lie on your back on a mat or carpeted surface. Hold one medium-to-heavy dumbbell in each hand directly over your chest, with your arms extended straight up and your palms facing your feet, so that you can see the backs of your hands. Bend your knees and hips 90 degrees, so your shins are in tabletop position parallel to the floor). Your knees should be over your hips and your navel pulled toward your spine. Slowly bend your elbows and lower your arms out to your sides, stopping just before the backs of your arms touch the floor. Hold for a moment. As you press your arms upward to the starting position, extend one leg, pressing out through the heel. Bend your elbows again and pull the knee back to the tabletop position. Repeat with the other leg. Alternate the chest press and leg press for 10 to 16 repetitions.

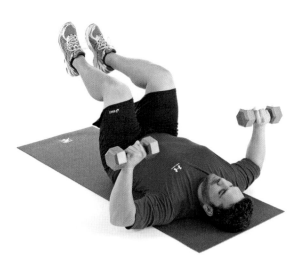

Tips

- Maintain a neutral spine and don't let your back arch as you bend your elbows or press your leg out.
- Keep your neck relaxed.
- Lower your leg as far only as you can control it.

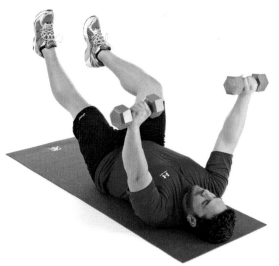

Intermediate Progression

Lower the extended leg closer to the floor.

Advanced Progression

Extend both legs to your point of control (but be sure to keep your core engaged and back neutral).

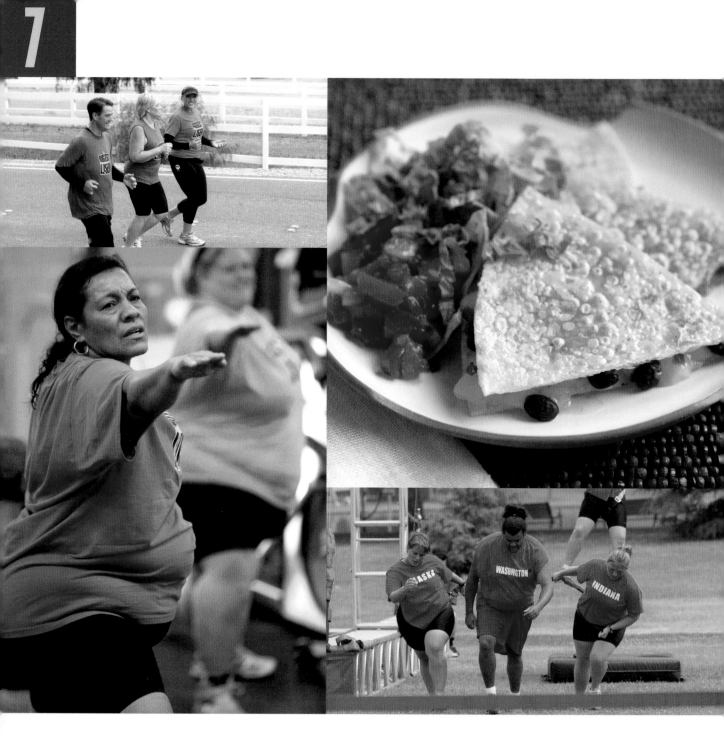

7

Week 4: Under Pressure

It's known as "the silent killer." High blood pressure may produce no noticeable symptoms and can be easily overlooked—but it can have a grave impact on your health. High blood pressure is not only a risk factor for heart disease but also can cause traumatic health crises, such as heart failure and stroke.

Blood pressure is interconnected with heart function and thus is a key indicator of overall health. It is crucial to know your blood pressure and work to maintain a healthy number through diet and lifestyle.

Season 6 contestant Jerry Skeabeck had the dubious distinction of being classified as one of the sickest cast members in the history of *The Biggest Loser.* Dr. Huizenga said that just thinking about Jerry kept him awake at night! When Jerry arrived at the Ranch, he was taking medicine for high blood pressure as well as a heart arrhythmia. After 6 weeks of exercise and healthy eating, the meds were gone.

"I think back to before *The Biggest Loser* and wonder, what the heck was I doing?" says Jerry today. "How could

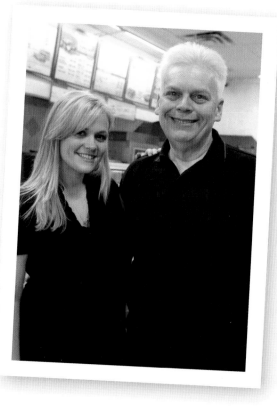

I have let my body get into that condition? I realized I had too many excuses, and I learned to just stop making them. I started my season at 380 pounds. With exercise and better eating habits, I was able to knock off 115 pounds for our season finale. The best part? My medical conditions are gone! Who would have thought I would ever feel this great?"

These days, Jerry says he feels better than ever. "I am much more confident in my everyday actions," he says. "I challenge myself continually to put myself first so I can be an asset to my family and friends. I love working with those who want to change their lives to be healthier. And it's great at age 53 to hear comments about how good my arms and chest look. People say, 'You must work out!'"

James Crutchfield of Season 9 says that high blood pressure landed him in the emergency room. "I had a 911 situation," he says. "My blood pressure was 190/130. I realized, at age 30, that medi-

cal problems had caught up with me. The 'invincibility' factor that came with being young disappeared. I realized I wouldn't live another year at that rate, much less another 10 or 20 years."

But after a few solid weeks of eating healthfully, exercising, and losing weight, James no longer needed medication to manage his high blood pressure. "I make sure to eat a low-sodium diet to combat high blood pressure," he says. "Organic foods with lots of vegetables and lean proteins help a lot. And I look for foods that contain powerful antioxidants."

James's twin brother and Season 9 teammate, John, has also experienced a radical change in his health. "My high blood pressure has been cured! I had all kinds of stomach and intestinal problems when I came to the Ranch, but now I'm medication free except for an over-the-counter antacid. No more prescriptions for me."

Season 8 winner Danny Cahill, also diagnosed with high blood pressure before he came to the

Alexandra White, Season 8

I used to exercise all the time, which is a shock because I was overweight. But one thing I never really did was push myself. You can't get complacent with workouts. Every week, it's time to take it up to a new level. Get uncomfortable. That uncomfortable feeling is always temporary, and at the end of the day you can look back and say, "I did that, I pushed myself." You'll feel better because of it.

Power Foods

Combat high blood pressure with:

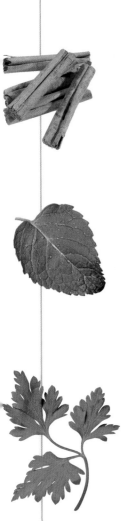

Low-sodium seasonings

- Cinnamon
- Cloves
- Cocoa powder (natural, unsweet-ened)
- Cumin
- Curry powder
- Dill
- Garlic
- Ginger
- Lavender
- Mint
- Mustard
- Onions
- Oregano
- Parsley
- Rosemary
- Saffron
- Sage
- Thyme
- Turmeric
- Vanilla

Potassium-rich fruits and vegetables

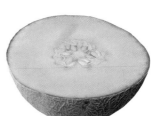

- Apricots
- Bananas
- Cantaloupe and honeydew melon
- Leafy greens
- Lima beans
- Mushrooms
- Peas
- Prunes
- Raisins and dates
- Spinach
- Sweet potatoes
- Tomatoes and low-sodium tomato sauce

Low-fat or fat-free dairy

- Cottage cheese
- Greek-style yogurt
- Ricotta cheese

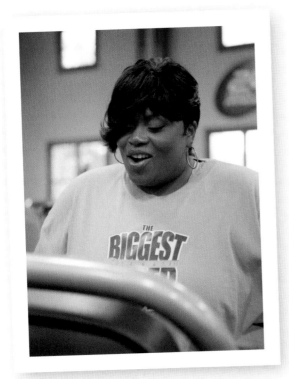

Ranch, no longer needed to take his blood pressure medication after 3 weeks on *The Biggest Loser* campus. "My high blood pressure is gone," he says, "and my edema is very minor! This new life is great. I can physically do things that were impossible before. I can run farther and faster than ever before in my life. My family is so happy. We do things outside together, and I can keep up with my kids! I actually wear them out! My wife is so happy—and she, too, has lost over 60 pounds."

For Carla Triplett of Season 7, it was "eye opening" to be diagnosed as having borderline high blood pressure at the age of 36. "I have a good friend who

had a mild stroke at 35, and I definitely did not want that to happen to me," says Carla. "But Dr. H assured me my hypertension was reversible.

"Life is too short," she adds. "You should live every day as if it's your last. Tomorrow is not promised. I wasted too many years not having fun, afraid of what people might say about me because of my weight. Not anymore. I've gained love and respect for myself. If I don't love myself first, nobody will love me like I deserve. I've gained confidence in knowing that I could lose 128 pounds on my own, without having surgery or taking diet pills. I realized weight loss is possible when you set your mind to it."

About High Blood Pressure

Blood pressure is a measure of the force of blood against the inside walls of your blood vessels. It is typically written or stated as two numbers:

Cheryl George, Season 9

I'm learning to be insistent in the grocery store. If I want some produce that's organic and I don't see it, I'm going to ask that they stock it.

THE BIGGES[T]

- The first or top number is the systolic pressure, representing the force of the blood as your heart muscle contracts (or "beats").
- The second or bottom number represents the pressure when the heart rests between beats. This is called diastolic pressure.

Throughout the course of the day, it's normal for blood pressure to rise and fall. But when blood pressure consistently stays high for too long, it is diagnosed as hypertension—the medical term for high blood pressure.

High blood pressure affects 31.3 percent of Americans. But without symptoms, high blood pressure often goes undetected; one in five people with high blood pressure don't know they have it. In this case, ignorance is definitely not bliss. As discussed in Chapter 5, high blood pressure is a major risk factor for heart disease, the leading cause of death in the United States.

In addition, high blood pressure can cause blood vessels to burst suddenly—which can result in a stroke. If blood vessels in the eyes rupture or burst from high blood pressure, impairment of sight, including total blindness, can result. High blood pressure can also thicken and narrow the blood vessels of the kidneys, blocking their ability to filter waste from the body.

Undiagnosed high blood pressure led to a severe stroke for Season 7 contestant Cathy Skell's grandmother when she was in her early 60s. "I was on high blood pressure medication for about 8 years," says Cathy. "My dosage was actually doubled about 1½ years ago, because my blood pressure was not stabilized.

"After I lost my first 30 pounds at the Ranch," Cathy continues, "Dr. H took me off my blood pressure meds. I was scared. I'm from Wisconsin—out in California at the Ranch it was 112 degrees! I was 49 years old, 263 pounds, and pushing myself to my physical limits in our workouts. I was afraid of having a heart attack or a stroke. Little did I know (or understand) what great care I was in! My

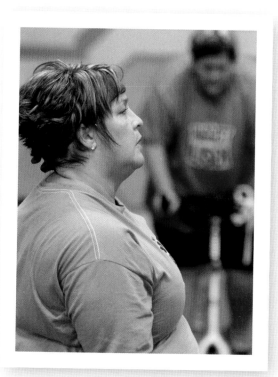

pulse and blood pressure were monitored all the time. After a few weeks, it was amazing how much my blood pressure had lowered. I ran my first half-marathon in September in under 3 hours. I am so proud of that accomplishment, considering I never tried or even thought to run in the past because of my asthma and high blood pressure."

Health care providers classify high blood pressure according to its cause. In most cases, high pressure doesn't have a single, specific treatable cause. This form is called essential hypertension. Rarely, the cause of high blood pressure is some other underlying condition, such as a kidney

disorder. This form is called secondary hypertension and may be temporary if the underlying cause is treated. Women may develop high blood pressure when they become pregnant, risking damage to their organs along with fetal complications.

Risk Factors

Several risk factors for high blood pressure are beyond your control. One is age: It's estimated that about 90 percent of middle-aged adults will develop high blood pressure in the remainder of their lifetimes.

For women, hormonal changes are another risk factor. Menopause is linked to higher blood pressure, which can be more pronounced than the elevated effect associated with weight gain (which often occurs around menopause). Additionally, a few women may experience elevated blood pressure in connection with hormone replacement therapy or the use of birth control pills.

Family history is an indicator of high blood pressure risk, and ethnicity can also be a factor. Season 3's Ken Coleman was inspired to apply for *The Biggest Loser* in part because his father died of hypertension. Ken was diagnosed with high blood pressure, too. But his symptoms disappeared after a few weeks on the Ranch. Today, Ken says he takes steps to keep his blood pressure under control and ensure it never soars too high again. "I watch

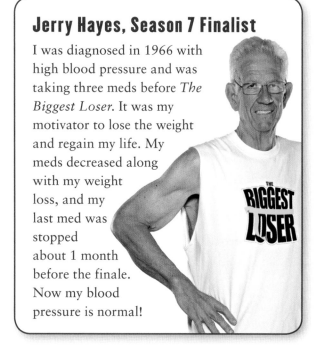

Jerry Hayes, Season 7 Finalist

I was diagnosed in 1966 with high blood pressure and was taking three meds before *The Biggest Loser*. It was my motivator to lose the weight and regain my life. My meds decreased along with my weight loss, and my last med was stopped about 1 month before the finale. Now my blood pressure is normal!

what I eat, and I pay careful attention to how my food is prepared, using spices instead of salt."

While you can't control your gender, genetics, or age, there are plenty of other risk factors that you *can* control.

What to Watch For: Understanding the Numbers

Because your blood pressure rises and falls throughout the day, your doctor will want to measure it several times on different days before making a diagnosis. NIH recommends the following criteria for determining whether your blood pressure falls within the healthy range:

- Normal: Systolic is less than 120, and diastolic is less than 80.
- Prehypertension: Systolic is between 120 and 139, and diastolic is between 80 and 89.
- High blood pressure: Systolic is 140 or higher, and diastolic is 90 or higher.

These numbers are valid only if you aren't already taking medications to lower your blood pressure and you don't have diabetes. If you do have diabetes, any measurement over 130/80 classifies as high blood pressure.

Especially for younger people, the diastolic number is an important indicator for hypertension. The higher the diastolic blood pressure, the greater the risk of heart attacks, strokes, and kidney failure.

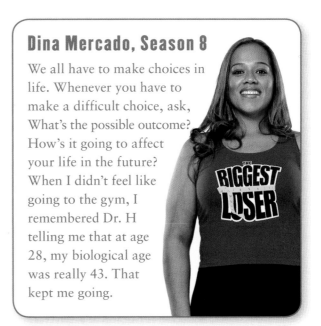

Dina Mercado, Season 8

We all have to make choices in life. Whenever you have to make a difficult choice, ask, What's the possible outcome? How's it going to affect your life in the future? When I didn't feel like going to the gym, I remembered Dr. H telling me that at age 28, my biological age was really 43. That kept me going.

As you age, the diastolic pressure begins to decrease and the systolic number starts to rise. When only the systolic pressure number is too high, the condition is called isolated systolic hypertension, or ISH. About 65 percent of people over age 60 with hypertension have ISH, making it the most common form of high blood pressure for older Americans.

Though optimal blood pressure is less than 120 systolic and less than 80 diastolic, you should be evaluated if your blood pressure is too low. Low blood pressure, known as hypotension, usually refers to a systolic/diastolic ratio of less than 90/60. Low blood pressure with accompanying symptoms such as lightheadedness or fainting could indicate an underlying medical condition.

The Weight-Loss Connection

The more you weigh, the more blood you need to feed your body's cells. As the amount of blood circulated through your blood vessels increases, so does the pressure on your artery walls. The epidemic of obesity in our country may be responsible for up to 30 percent of the hypertension in Americans. Additionally, people who are obese are twice as likely to develop high blood pressure as those at a healthy weight. If you're overweight, losing just 10 pounds can help reduce your blood pressure.

Comprehensive research shows that dietary and lifestyle changes don't just control weight: The changes can help to lower blood pressure. Scientists supported by the National Heart, Lung, and Blood Institute of NIH conducted two major studies, both of which showed that blood pressure can be reduced by following many of the principles outlined in this book. The researchers developed an eating plan called DASH (Dietary Approaches to Stop Hypertension), which is low in saturated fat, cholesterol, and total fat and recommends consuming fruits, vegetables, and fat-free or low-fat milk and milk products—as does *The Biggest Loser* eating plan.

Slash the Salt

To control blood pressure, aim to consume no more than 2,400 milligrams of sodium each day. Getting fewer than 1,500 milligrams daily, or the equivalent of about ⅔ teaspoon of table salt, is

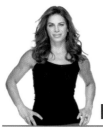

Biggest Loser Trainer Tip: Jillian Michaels

If you're serious about weight loss, here's a critical tip: Keep a food journal. Write down every calorie consumed. It'll hold you accountable for all your food and beverage choices. It's been reported that keeping a food journal can actually *double* your weight loss. So grab a notepad, write everything down, and use your *Biggest Loser* calorie book to find the calorie count of each item. As long as you burn more calories than you've taken in, you'll be sure to lose weight.

even better. Of course, most of the sodium in the American diet doesn't come from a saltshaker but from processed foods or cooking methods high in salt content. To reduce sodium:

- **Limit processed foods.** Salt is a preservative, so many packaged foods contain high amounts of sodium. Cut back on frozen dinners, pizza, packaged mixes, canned soups or broths, and salad dressings; opt instead for fresh foods and whole grains. If you do buy processed foods:
  - Check the label carefully. "Low sodium" only means that the food contains half the sodium of the original—the sodium content may still be high.
  - Opt for plain frozen vegetables or canned versions labeled "no salt added."
  - Rinse canned foods to remove some sodium.
  - Choose ready-to-eat breakfast cereals that are low in sodium.

- **Leave the saltshaker in the cabinet.** Instead, try flavoring your foods with the antioxidant-rich herbs and spices listed on page 161. They'll add zing to your food without extra sodium.

Additionally, avoid seasoning mixes, which are often high in sodium unless otherwise noted.

- **Cook rice, pasta, and hot cereal without salt.** The instructions on the packages of these foods usually suggest you add salt, but it is not neces-sary. Also, cut back on instant or flavored rice, pasta, and cereal mixes, which usually contain added salt (and less fiber) than the slower-to-cook versions.

Boost Potassium

Potassium is a mineral that causes you to excrete sodium. If you have too little potassium in your system, you'll retain sodium. Potassium also plays an important role in muscle contraction; since your heart is one big muscle, this nutrient is essential for optimal heart health. The NIH Recommended Daily Intake of potassium for an average adult is about 4,700 milligrams. Keep in mind, though, that too much potassium can be harmful, as it affects the balance of fluids in the body. If your potassium is low, focus first on adding the mineral through dietary sources, not supplements, and consult your doctor. The fruits and vegetables listed in the chart on page 161 are rich in potassium and can easily be incorporated into your diet.

Don't Skip the Dairy

Aim for two to three servings of low-fat or fat-free dairy products each day. Large-scale studies have found that people who eat a lot of calcium have lower blood pressure than those who get less of this nutrient. Eating low-fat dairy as well as plenty of fruits and vegetables, along with cutting back on saturated and total fat, may reduce your systolic blood pressure by 8 to 14 points!

Quaff Green Tea; Sip Coffee

Drinking a cup of antioxidant-rich green tea every day offers many health benefits—and may lower blood pressure. A 2004 study found that people who drank 4 to 20 ounces of green or oolong tea daily were 46 percent less likely to have hypertension.

Coffee, on the other hand, is a different story. It remains unclear whether caffeine raises blood pressure over the long term, but it may increase blood pressure temporarily, especially in people who are not habitual coffee or caffeinated-beverage drinkers. Caffeine can also raise your heart rate and blood pressure during exercise. There's no harm in 1 or 2 cups of coffee each day, according to the AHA, but if you normally drink more than that, cut back.

Let Off Steam

The "fight-or-flight" reaction to stress releases a surge of adrenaline and cortisol intended to help you react quickly to imminent danger—a response hardwired from ancient times, when stress was caused by animal predators rather than work deadlines. High levels of stress can lead to a temporary spike in blood pressure; prolonged stress can contribute to elevated cholesterol, increased blood clotting, and atherosclerosis—which, along with high blood pressure, contribute to heart disease.

Reducing stress, then, is a worthy goal for keeping blood pressure and heart disease in check. But if you try to relax by eating more, you're being counterproductive. And smoking cigarettes actually causes a further spike in your blood pressure!

Instead, aim to reduce stress naturally by treating your body right.

- **Get plenty of sleep.** Lack of sleep taxes your body, so be disciplined and treat yourself to this luxury, whether it's napping during the day or going to bed earlier.
- **Practice stress relief.** Regular prayer, meditation, guided visualization (which is like organized daydreaming), and deep breathing have powerful relaxation qualities. Making time to do one of these relaxation techniques can help lower your stress levels in general and, when you're caught up in a stressful situation, allow you to quickly regain a sense of control.
- **Get moving.** People who are inactive tend to

have higher heart rates. This means your heart must work harder with each contraction—and exert more force on your blood vessels, resulting in higher blood pressure. Getting at least 30 minutes of exercise per day is a good way to reduce blood pressure. Engaging in a physical activity you enjoy—such as playing touch football, swimming, dancing, or practicing yoga—provides the added benefit of reducing stress.

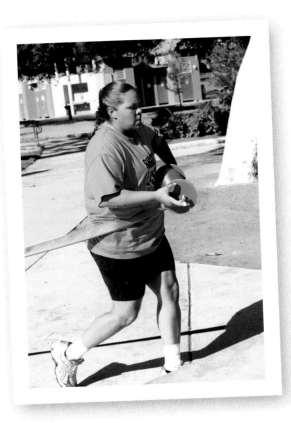

Making the Change

Now that Season 6's Jerry Skeabeck is leading a happy, healthy life, free of the complications of high blood pressure, he wants to encourage others to do the same.

"I believe we are all capable of making these changes in our lives. We have to question how badly we want it. Are we ready to put a plan together for exercise and nutrition and stick to it? Negative people get negative results. Surround yourself with positive attitudes. You will find that this will make it easier to start working toward your goals. Most people will find the results addictive, from working out in the gym to the changes they make in their eating habits. I'm a convert to health!"

Week 4 Menu Plan

MONDAY   1,535 calories

Breakfast

½ cup diced watermelon

Omelet: 3 egg whites, 2 tablespoons diced tomato, 1 teaspoon chopped dill, 2 tablespoons low-fat feta cheese, and 1 cup chopped baby spinach

Small quesadilla made with ½ small corn tortilla and 1 tablespoon low-fat Jack cheese

Iced tea with fresh lemon

Snack

½ cup fat-free vanilla yogurt with 1 sliced apple and 1 tablespoon chopped walnuts

Lunch

Chicken salad: 4 ounces diced grilled chicken, 2 cups chopped romaine lettuce, ½ cup halved cherry tomatoes, 1 diced hard-boiled egg, 1 tablespoon chopped basil, 2 tablespoons diced bell pepper, and 2 tablespoons low-fat vinaigrette

2 Wasa whole grain crackers

1 medium nectarine

Iced tea with lime

Snack

2 spears grilled or cooked asparagus wrapped in 1 ounce lox or smoked salmon

Dinner

4 ounces shrimp grilled or sautéed with 1 teaspoon olive oil and 1 teaspoon chopped garlic

1 medium artichoke, steamed

½ cup whole wheat couscous with 2 tablespoons diced bell pepper, ¼ cup chickpeas, 1 teaspoon chopped cilantro, and 1 tablespoon fat-free honey-mustard vinaigrette

½ cup sliced strawberries with ½ cup fat-free vanilla frozen yogurt

Green tea

TUESDAY   1,495 calories

Breakfast

Breakfast frittata: 3 large egg whites (½ cup), 2 tablespoons diced bell peppers, 2 tablespoons chopped spinach, 2 tablespoons shredded low-fat provolone cheese, and 2 teaspoons pesto

½ cup fresh raspberries

1 **Banana-Berry Muffin** (page 176)

1 cup fat-free milk

Snack

½ cup low-fat vanilla yogurt with 1 tablespoon ground flaxseed and ½ cup diced peach or pear

Lunch

Portobello pizzas: 2 portobello mushroom caps, each filled with 2 tablespoons low-fat marinara sauce, 2 tablespoons crumbled cooked lean turkey sausage, and 1 tablespoon shredded low-fat mozzarella cheese and baked at 400°F for approximately 10 minutes

Tomato-cucumber salad: 5 slices fresh tomato, ¼ cup sliced cucumber, 1 teaspoon chopped fresh thyme, and 1 tablespoon fat-free Italian dressing

1 medium orange

Iced tea

Snack

Smoothie: ¾ cup fat-free milk; ½ banana; ½ cup plain, fat-free Greek-style yogurt; and ¼ cup sliced strawberries

Dinner

4 ounces red snapper baked with 1 teaspoon olive oil, 1 teaspoon lemon juice, and ½ teaspoon sodium-free seasoning

1 cup spaghetti squash with 1 teaspoon olive oil and 2 teaspoons grated Parmesan cheese

1 cup steamed green beans sprinkled with 1 tablespoon slivered almonds

Sparkling water with lemon

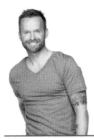

Biggest Loser Trainer Tip: Bob Harper

I hear it all the time. Reading food labels can be confusing. But it doesn't have to be. There are three important things to look for to start losing weight and living healthy. First is serving size. Just because a food is in one package does not mean it's just one meal. Then calories: Keeping track of calories consumed is the most important thing *The Biggest Loser* contestants do every day. Finally, you should not exceed your daily values for fat, cholesterol, and sodium. Don't be afraid of the food label. Let it be your guide to a healthy lifestyle.

WEDNESDAY   1,545 calories

Breakfast

1 cup low-sodium tomato vegetable juice

3 egg whites (½ cup) scrambled with
  1 teaspoon chopped cilantro, ¼ cup chopped
  red onion, ¼ cup sliced mushrooms, and
  1 tablespoon shredded low-fat Cheddar
  cheese

2 links lean turkey breakfast sausage

1 cup fresh blueberries

Green tea

Snack

8 triangles whole wheat pita chips and
  2 tablespoons hummus

Lunch

Chicken Caesar salad: 4 ounces boneless,
  skinless roast chicken; 1 cup chopped
  romaine lettuce; ½ cup sliced bell pepper;
  ¼ cup chopped scallions; and 2 tablespoons
  low-fat Caesar dressing

Herbal tea

Snack

½ cup fat-free cottage cheese with ½ cup
  tomato salsa

Dinner

4-ounce salmon burger, grilled

1 cup oven-roasted cauliflower and broccoli
  florets

¾ cup cooked brown rice

1 cup watercress salad with 1 tablespoon light
  balsamic vinaigrette

½ cup fat-free ricotta with ½ cup raspberries
  and 1 tablespoon chopped almonds

Ice water with lemon

THURSDAY   1,515 calories

Breakfast

Frittata: 3 large egg whites, 2 tablespoons
  diced roasted bell peppers, 2 teaspoons
  chopped spinach, 2 tablespoons shredded
  reduced-fat mozzarella cheese, and
  2 teaspoons chopped basil

½ cup fresh raspberries

O'Neal Hampton, Season 9

Educate yourself about healthy cooking. On the Ranch, we have
nutritionist Cheryl Forberg to take us grocery shopping and teach us
how to cook. But at home, pick up magazines that have healthy
recipes; watch healthy cooking shows on TV. Look up healthy recipes
online. The information is all around you.

1 small bran muffin

1 cup fat-free milk

Snack

½ cup low-fat vanilla yogurt with 1 tablespoon ground flaxseed and ½ cup diced pear

Lunch

4 ounces sliced turkey breast

Tomato-cucumber salad: 5 slices tomato, ¼ cup sliced cucumber, 1 teaspoon chopped fresh thyme, and 1 tablespoon fat-free Italian dressing

1 medium orange

Snack

Smoothie: ¾ cup fat-free milk, ½ banana, ½ cup low-fat yogurt, and ¼ cup raspberries

Dinner

4 ounces red snapper baked with 1 teaspoon olive oil, 1 teaspoon lemon juice, and ½ teaspoon sodium-free seasoning

1 cup spaghetti squash with 1 teaspoon olive oil and 2 teaspoons grated Parmesan cheese

1 cup steamed green beans with 1 tablespoon slivered almonds

FRIDAY   1,485 calories

Breakfast

¼ cup old-fashioned oatmeal (cooked with water) topped with 1 tablespoon chopped pumpkin seeds

Omelet: 1 egg and 2 egg whites, fresh dill or other herbs, and 1 ounce feta cheese

1 kiwifruit, sliced

Green tea or water

Snack

½ turkey sandwich made with 2 ounces lean turkey, 1 tomato slice, 1 lettuce leaf, and 1 teaspoon Dijon mustard on 1 slice whole grain bread

Lunch

5-ounce salmon burger, grilled, on whole grain bun with 1 tomato slice, lettuce, and 1 teaspoon Dijon mustard

1 apple

1 cup fat-free milk

Snack

Kefir or yogurt smoothie: 6 ounces unsweetened kefir or fat-free yogurt, ¼ cup mixed berries, and 1 teaspoon ground flaxseed

Green tea or water

Dinner

1 serving **White Chicken Chili** (page 179)

Green salad: 2 cups baby spinach or mixed greens; 5 cherry tomatoes, halved; and 1 tablespoon low-fat vinaigrette

1 pear

Water

SATURDAY   1,525 calories

Breakfast

½ cup fat-free ricotta cheese topped with 1 tablespoon ground flaxseed and ¼ cup fresh berries

¼ cup old-fashioned oatmeal (cooked with water) and ½ teaspoon ground cinnamon

1 soft-boiled egg

1 cup fat-free milk

Green tea or water

Snack

1 large apple with 1 tablespoon almond butter or peanut butter

Lunch

1 serving **Grilled Prawn Salad with Tomatoes and Avocado Aioli** (page 181)

1 kiwifruit, sliced

1 cup fat-free milk

Snack

1 hard-boiled egg

1 apple

3 walnuts

Dinner

1 serving **Black Bean Quesadillas** (page 182)

2" wedge cantaloupe

1 cup water

Green tea

SUNDAY   1,495 calories

Breakfast

Yogurt parfait: 6 ounces plain, fat-free Greek-style yogurt; 1 tablespoon ground flaxseed; ¼ cup mixed berries; and ¼ cup Kashi GoLean cereal

Omelet: 1 egg, 2 egg whites, and fresh herbs

Green tea or water

Snack

Chicken quesadilla: 2 tablespoons grated pepper Jack cheese and 1½ ounces roasted turkey breast or chicken on 1 corn tortilla

Lunch

Greek salad: 4 ounces grilled chicken, 2 cups chopped romaine lettuce, ¼ cup diced cucumber, ¼ cup diced red bell pepper, 2 tablespoons chopped scallion, 2 tablespoons crumbled low-fat feta cheese, and 1 tablespoon low-fat Caesar dressing

½ cup fat-free vanilla yogurt with 1 tablespoon chopped dates and 1 tablespoon chopped pecans

Iced tea

Snack

½ cup cottage cheese topped with 1 tablespoon ground flaxseed

1 pear

Water

Dinner

1 cup low-fat lentil or black bean soup topped with 1 tablespoon plain, fat-free Greek-style yogurt and 1 teaspoon chopped chives or scallion

1 cup dark green leafy salad with 6 ounces grilled halibut

½ cup alfalfa sprouts and 1 tablespoon low-fat balsamic dressing

1 cup fat-free milk

BANANA-BERRY MUFFINS

These moist, delicious muffins are a great replacement for the calorie bombs sold at most bakeries and cafés. Sweet and satisfying, Banana-Berry Muffins are loaded with antioxidants and fiber. Make a few batches at once and store in the freezer until needed.

1½   **cups unprocessed wheat bran or oat bran**

1   **cup white whole wheat flour**

2   **tablespoons ground flaxseed (see note)**

1¼   **teaspoons baking soda**

1   **teaspoon ground cinnamon**

⅛   **teaspoon salt**

¾   **cup unsweetened vanilla almond milk or fat-free milk**

¼   **cup agave nectar or dark honey**

2   **ripe medium bananas, mashed with a fork**

1   **large egg**

2   **tablespoons olive oil**

1   **teaspoon vanilla extract**

1   **cup fresh (or frozen) blueberries**

½   **cup pitted chopped prunes (optional)**

Position a rack in the center of the oven and preheat the oven to 400°F. Lightly coat a nonstick 12-cup muffin pan with cooking oil spray.

In a medium bowl, combine the bran, flour, flaxseed, baking soda, cinnamon, and salt. Set aside. In another medium bowl or in a blender, combine the milk, agave nectar or honey, bananas, egg, oil, and vanilla until smooth.

Make a well in the center of the dry ingredients and pour in ⅓ of the liquid mixture. Using a spoon, stir until smooth. Add the remaining liquid mixture and stir just until combined. Add the blueberries and prunes, if desired; stir again, but do not overmix.

Spoon ¼ cup batter into each prepared muffin cup. Bake for about 14 minutes, or until the tops spring back when pressed gently in the centers. Do not overbake. Cool in the pan on a wire rack for 10 minutes before removing the muffins from the pan. Serve warm, or cool completely on the rack.

Note: If you can't find ground flaxseed in your local health food store, you can grind whole flaxseeds in a clean spice grinder to the consistency of cornmeal.

Makes 12 (1-muffin) servings

Per serving: 140 calories, 4 g protein, 25 g carbohydrates (10 g sugars), 4 g fat (0 g saturated), 20 mg cholesterol, 6 g fiber, 170 mg sodium

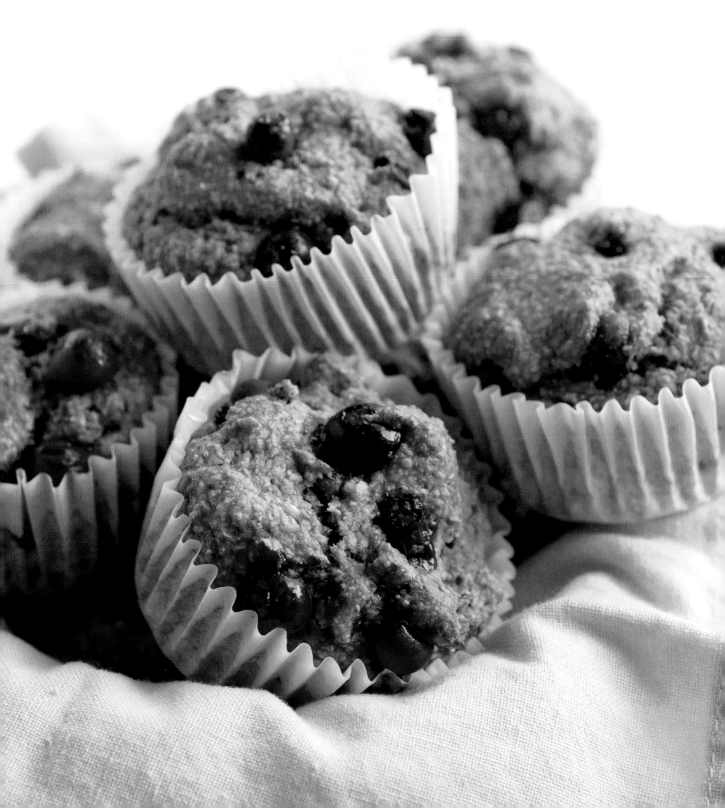

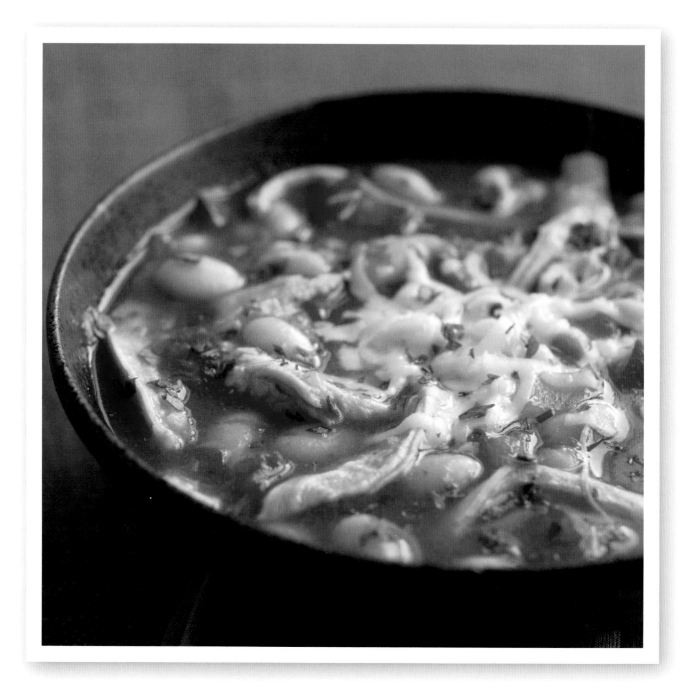

WHITE CHICKEN CHILI

Season 7 contestant Kristin Steede introduced me to this variation on a traditional tomato-based chili, and it's become one of my favorites. You can substitute turkey breast or lean pork loin for the chicken and swap in your favorite beans for endless variations. This recipe is quick and easy, and the chili keeps well in the freezer.

1 pound boneless, skinless chicken or turkey breast or 1 pound lean pork tenderloin

4½ cups cooked great northern beans

2 cups fat-free, low-sodium chicken broth

2 cups thick and chunky salsa

1 cup reduced-fat mozzarella cheese

Chopped cilantro (optional)

Cook and shred the chicken or turkey breast or dice the tenderloin; set aside. In a large saucepan, mix together the beans, broth, and salsa. Heat through and add extra broth, if desired. Stir in the meat and cheese and top with cilantro, if desired. Serve hot.

Makes about 8 (1-cup) servings

Per serving: **230 calories, 26 g protein, 24 g carbohydrates (0 g sugars), 4 g fat (2 g saturated), 30 mg cholesterol, 8 g fiber, 230 mg sodium**

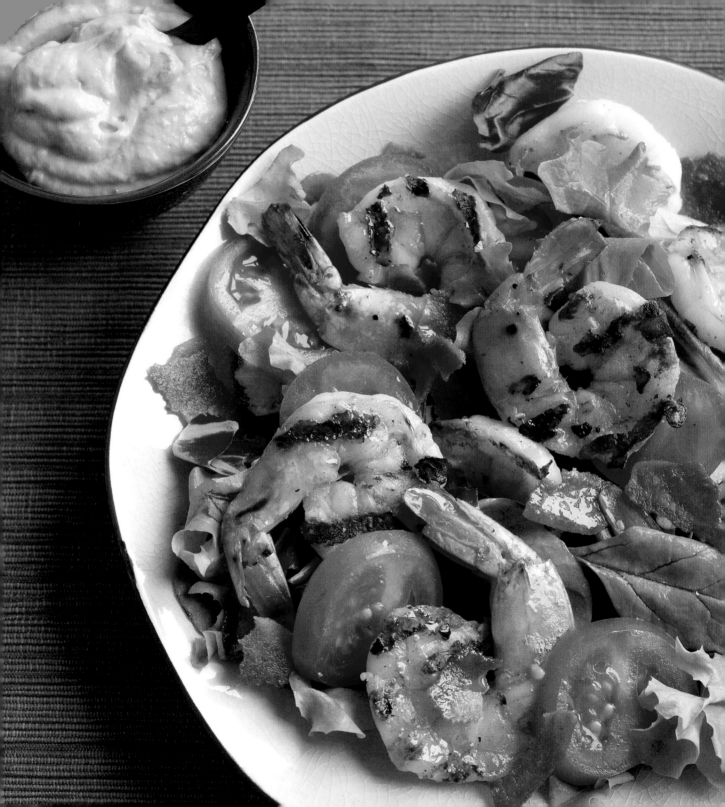

GRILLED PRAWN SALAD WITH TOMATOES AND AVOCADO AIOLI

Prawns are similar to shrimp but are a bit larger in size. If you can't find prawns at your local grocery store or fish market, you can use fresh or frozen jumbo shrimp. This salad provides plenty of potassium, folate, and heart-healthy fats. It makes for a delicious light lunch, especially in the summer months.

---

8 large fresh prawns, peeled and deveined

2 teaspoons extra-virgin olive oil

½ teaspoon crushed garlic

4 slices (2 ounces) lean turkey bacon

4 cups mixed salad greens

2 Roma tomatoes, sliced lengthwise

4 tablespoons Avocado Aioli (below)

Season the prawns with the oil and garlic. Cover and refrigerate for at least 1 hour.

Heat a grill or nonstick skillet to medium high. Cook the bacon until crisp. Drain on a paper towel. Grill or sauté the prawns for about 1 minute on each side, until pink. Drain on a paper towel until cool enough to handle and cut in half lengthwise.

Layer the greens with the prawns, bacon, and sliced tomatoes. Top each salad with a 2-tablespoon dollop of Avocado Aioli.

Makes 2 servings

Per serving: 140 calories, 14 g protein, 6 g carbohydrates (2 g sugars), 8 g fat (1 g saturated), 79 mg cholesterol, 3 g fiber, 200 mg sodium

AVOCADO AIOLI

This creamy, garlicky spread is delicious on sandwiches or as a dip for fresh veggies.

---

1 medium very ripe avocado

⅓ cup plain, fat-free Greek-style yogurt

1 tablespoon chopped basil

2 teaspoons minced garlic

1 teaspoon fresh lemon juice

½ teaspoon salt

¼ teaspoon ground black pepper

Combine the avocado, yogurt, basil, garlic, lemon juice, salt, and black pepper in a food processor and process until just smooth. Use immediately or store in the refrigerator.

Makes about 1 cup, or 8 (2-tablespoon) servings

Per serving: 35 calories, 2 g protein, 2 g carbohydrates (0 g sugars), 4 g fat (0 g saturated), 0 mg cholesterol, 1 g fiber, 150 mg sodium

BLACK BEAN QUESADILLAS

This is one of Season 8 winner Danny Cahill's favorite meals, especially since it's what his wife, Darci, prepared for him the first day he came home from the Ranch! The beans, salsa, and cheese give these quesadillas all the flavor and texture you crave from rich Mexican food, with only 6 grams of fat per serving.

2 brown rice tortillas (burrito size)

2 slices reduced-fat pepper Jack cheese

½ cup black beans

¼ cup fresh salsa

2 cups shredded romaine lettuce

Spray a large nonstick skillet with cooking oil spray and heat over medium heat.

One at a time, warm each tortilla on both sides. Leave the second tortilla in the pan and tear the cheese into pieces to cover the tortilla in a single layer. Spread the beans over the tortilla and heat for 1 to 2 minutes. Add the second tortilla and heat for 1 minute longer. Turn the quesadilla over and heat until the cheese is just melted.

Remove the quesadilla from the pan and cut into 6 triangles. Place 3 triangles on a plate and top with salsa and lettuce.

Makes 2 servings

Per serving: 240 calories, 10 g protein, 38 g carbohydrates (1 g sugars), 6 g fat (2 g saturated), 10 mg cholesterol, 7 g fiber, 290 mg sodium

Liz Young, Season 8

You can't eat your emotions, or they'll eat you up inside. Learn to put your issues on the table and talk about them. The better care you take of yourself, the more you're going to realize that you're worth it. You deserve a good life.

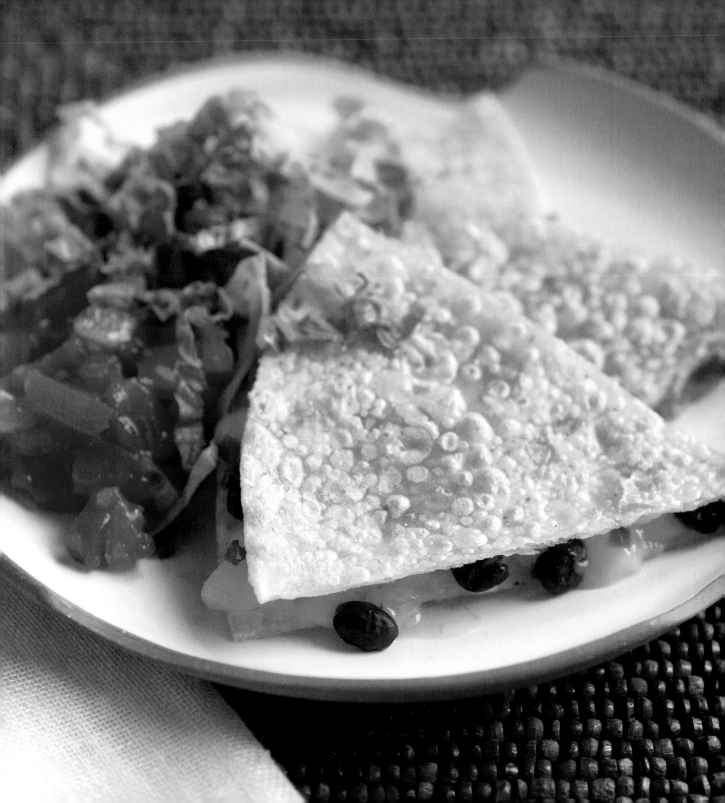

Week 4 Exercises

When you improve your fitness level, you can lower your blood pressure and possibly eliminate medications. Not only does regular exercise help maintain a healthy body weight, it also builds a strong heart that more easily pumps blood throughout the body, putting less stress on the arteries. The key here is getting *regular* exercise and making fitness a part of your lifestyle.

If you already have high blood pressure, you will need to get clearance for exercise from your doctor. Start your new routine slowly. Monitoring your progress and your blood pressure is imperative for two main reasons:

- It allows you to determine whether your exercise program is helping to lower your blood pressure.
- It will help you determine (along with the advice of your doctor) whether you need to reduce any blood pressure medication you are taking.

Decrease exercise intensity or consult your doctor if you have pain or pressure in your chest, arm, or jaw; experience dizziness or fatigue; or experience irregular heartbeat or shortness of breath.

Any of the workouts from weeks 1 through 3 are appropriate for the prevention and control of high blood pressure. However, to mix it up and add variety to your exercise program, this week we will focus on cardio and strength circuit training. This type of training develops aerobic and muscular conditioning simultaneously and provides up to double the calorie burn—making it an efficient use of time. In addition, variety helps prevent overuse injuries—and boredom!

Focus: Cardio/Strength Circuit Training
Workout Guidelines

- For this program, you will need an exercise band or tubing with handles. If you don't have tubing, you can substitute dumbbells. Tubing is ideal, as it offers a different type of resistance (generally of less intensity) and makes it easier to transition from strength to cardio exercises, because you don't have to put the band down.

- Remember to breathe! This may sound like a no-brainer, but be sure you inhale and exhale fully as you exercise. Holding your breath, especially during the resistance exercises, can elevate your blood pressure.

- Warm up for 5 minutes by marching in place or walking.

- Perform the tubing resistance exercises featured here for 15 to 20 repetitions and alternate basic cardio moves (jogging in place, high knees, jumping jacks, skaters).

- Begin with one circuit of each resistance and cardio exercise for a 20-minute workout (30 including warmup and stretching) and build up to two circuits for a 40-minute workout (50 including warmup and stretching).

- Follow this cardio workout with a gentle stretch for your legs, back, and chest, as well as your triceps and shoulders.

- For a well-rounded program, try this workout for 2 to 3 days a week in addition to cardio training 3 or 4 days a week. Alternate cardio and circuit days.

Mo DeWalt, Season 8

If you want to avoid high blood pressure, you'll have to start exercising. One day, you're not going to feel like going to the gym, but don't find excuses. Find reasons to do it. The reason to exercise is you want to be healthy. You want to live longer. Your loved ones need to see you around a lot longer than they're going to if you don't go to the gym.

REAR FLY

Begin by holding the handle of the tubing in each hand. Step on the tubing with one foot and hinge forward from the hips with knees slightly bent. Keeping your spine neutral and your abdominals engaged, pull the handles up and out to the sides of your body, squeezing the muscles in your upper back and midback. Hold for a moment, then release the tubing back down toward the floor. Repeat. After completing the recommended repetitions, follow up with 1 minute of cardio before moving onto the next exercise.

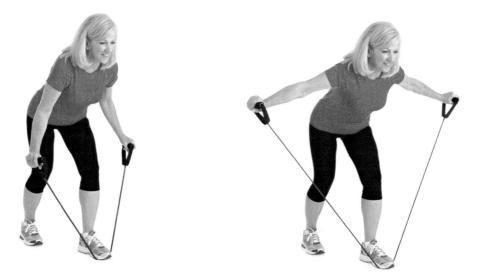

Tips

- Avoid rounding your back.
- Control the movement and don't allow your elbows to lock on the downward motion of the exercise.
- Keep your navel pulled in at all times.
- Keep your arms in line with your shoulders as you lift to the side. Don't allow your shoulders to hunch up to your ears.

Intermediate Progression

Change to a higher-resistance band or choke up on the tubing by wrapping it once around each hand. This creates more resistance.

Advanced Progression

Lift the back leg to challenge balance.

STATIONARY LUNGE

Begin in a staggered stance, with your left leg forward and your right leg back, heel off the floor. Place the tubing under your left foot and hold the handles at your hips or shoulders. Keeping your spine neutral, your shoulders over your hips, and your abdominals engaged, bend both knees until your left thigh is parallel to the floor and your right knee is a few inches off the floor. Hold for a moment, then straighten both legs. Repeat. After completing the recommended repetitions, follow up with 1 minute of cardio before moving onto the next exercise.

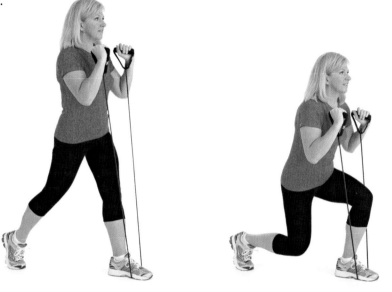

Tips

- Avoid rounding or arching your back.
- Keep your navel pulled in at all times.
- In the lunge, keep your left shin perpendicular to the floor so that your knee is directly over your ankle.
- Don't let your left knee move past your toes.

Intermediate Progression

Choke up on the tubing to create more resistance.

Advanced Progression

Add an overhead press as you lunge.

Note: Be sure to repeat on the other leg after completing 1 minute of cardio to continue the circuit.

CHEST PRESS

Stand with your feet a little wider than hip-width apart. Take the tubing around your midback and grab the handles with each hand so that the tubing is under your armpits. If the tubing is too long, double up the tubing so both handles are in your right hand. Inhale deeply, and as you exhale, press both arms forward, keeping your chest lifted and your navel pulled to your spine. Slowly bend your elbows and bring the tubing back toward your armpits. Repeat. After completing the recommended repetitions, follow up with 1 minute of cardio before moving onto the next exercise.

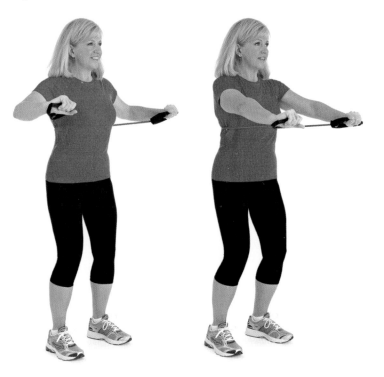

Tips

- Avoid arching your back or letting your chest cave in.
- Control the movement and don't allow your elbows to lock as you press out.
- Keep your navel pulled in at all times.
- Keep your wrists in line with your elbows and slightly below your shoulders.

Intermediate Progression

Choke up on the tubing to create more resistance.

Advanced Progression

Add an alternating front lunge.

BICEPS CURL

Hold a handle of the tubing in each hand. Step on the tubing in a narrow stance and hold the handles by your thighs, with your palms forward. Draw your navel to your spine, roll your shoulders back and down, and soften your knees. Slowly bend your elbows and bring the handles of the tubing up to your shoulders. Squeeze your biceps, then slowly return the handles to the starting position. Repeat. After completing the recommended repetitions, follow up with 1 minute of cardio before moving onto the next exercise.

Tips

- Avoid arching your back or letting your chest cave in.
- Control the movement and don't allow your elbows to lock as you extend your arms.
- Keep your navel pulled in at all times.
- Keep your elbows slightly in front of your torso.

Intermediate Progression

Choke up on the tubing to create more resistance.

Advanced Progression

Stand on one leg to challenge your balance.

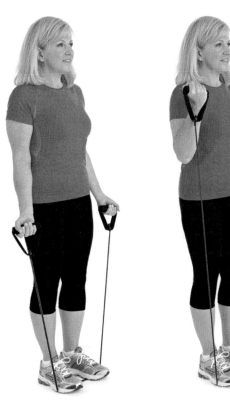

SQUAT

Hold a handle of the tubing in each hand. Step on the tubing with your feet a little wider than hip-width apart and hold the handles at your hips or shoulders. Draw your navel toward your spine, roll your shoulders back, and lengthen your spine. Send your hips back and bend your knees as if you were sitting in a chair, until your thighs are parallel to the floor. Push into your heels and return to standing. Repeat. After completing the recommended repetitions, follow up with 1 minute of cardio before moving onto the next exercise.

Tips

- Maintain your natural lower-back arch; avoiding rounding your back.
- Keep your focus forward.
- Keep your toes pointing forward.

Intermediate Progression

Choke up on the tubing to create more resistance.

Advanced Progression

Change to a single-leg squat.

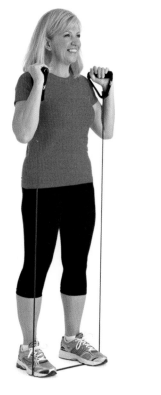
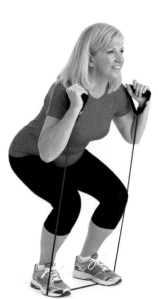

TRICEPS OVERHEAD EXTENSION

Hold one end of the tubing in your right hand and step on the other end with your left foot so that the tubing is on the inside of your leg. Step your right foot forward in a staggered stance, with the right knee bent. Bring the tubing handle in your right hand behind your back. Extend your left arm over your head, then bend both elbows and grab the handle with both hands. Pull your navel in and drop your shoulders away from your ears. Keeping your upper arms close to your head, straighten your arms until your elbows are extended. Hold for a moment, then bend your elbows and lower your hands behind your head. Repeat. After completing the recommended repetitions, follow up with 1 minute of cardio before moving onto the next exercise.

Tips

- Don't let your lower back arch or your ribs press out. Keep your core engaged.
- Maintain knee-over-ankle alignment of your front leg.
- Press your arms up, not forward.

Intermediate Progression

Shorten the length of the tubing by having more on the floor.

Advanced Progression

Add a lunge as you press up.

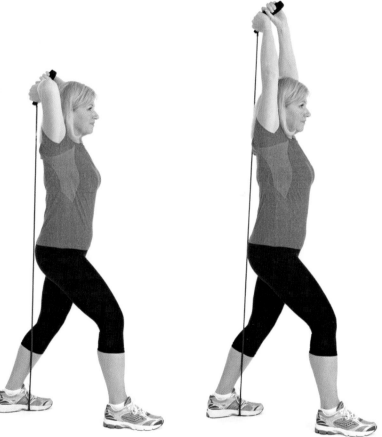

BUTT BLASTER

Begin on your hands and knees on a mat or carpeted surface. Slide your right foot through one tubing handle (like a stirrup); hold the other end on the floor with your right hand. Make sure there is no slack in the tubing and that the tubing is on the outside of your right leg. Keeping your spine neutral and core engaged, press your right leg back so that your knee is extended and your leg is parallel to the floor. Hold for a moment, then slowly bend your knee back in toward your chest. Repeat. After completing the recommended repetitions, follow up with 1 minute of cardio before moving onto the next exercise.

Tips

- Don't allow your back to round or arch.
- Press away from the floor with your arms to stabilize your shoulder girdle.
- Flex your foot and press out through your heel.
- To make it easier, lengthen the tubing to reduce the resistance.

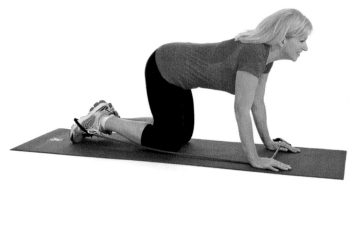

Intermediate Progression

Tighten up on the tubing.

Advanced Progression

Lift the leg higher, extending your hip, after you press back.

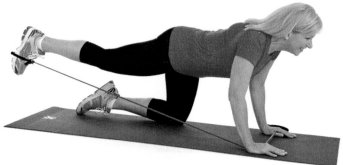

Note: Be sure to repeat on the other leg after completing 1 minute of cardio to continue the circuit.

LATERAL RAISE

Hold a handle of the tubing in each hand. Step on the tubing in a narrow stance and hold the handles next to your thighs. Draw your navel to your spine, roll your shoulders back and down, and soften your knees. Slowly lift your arms out to the sides with your elbows slightly bent. Hold for a moment, relax your neck, and then slowly return the tubing to the starting position. Repeat. After completing the recommended repetitions, follow up with 1 minute of cardio, and then stretch.

Tips

- Avoid arching your back or letting your chest cave in.
- Control the movement and don't allow the tubing to pull your arms down.
- Keep your navel pulled in at all times.
- Keep your shoulders down and away from your ears, and hold your elbows slightly higher than your wrists.

Intermediate Progression

Cross the tubing to create more resistance.

Advanced Progression

Stand on one leg to challenge balance.

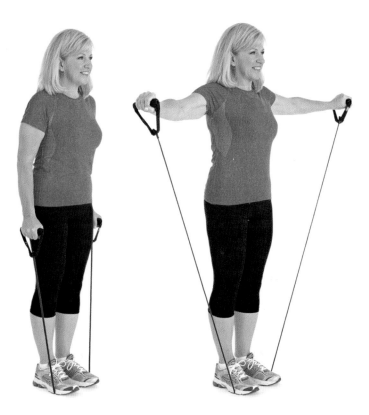

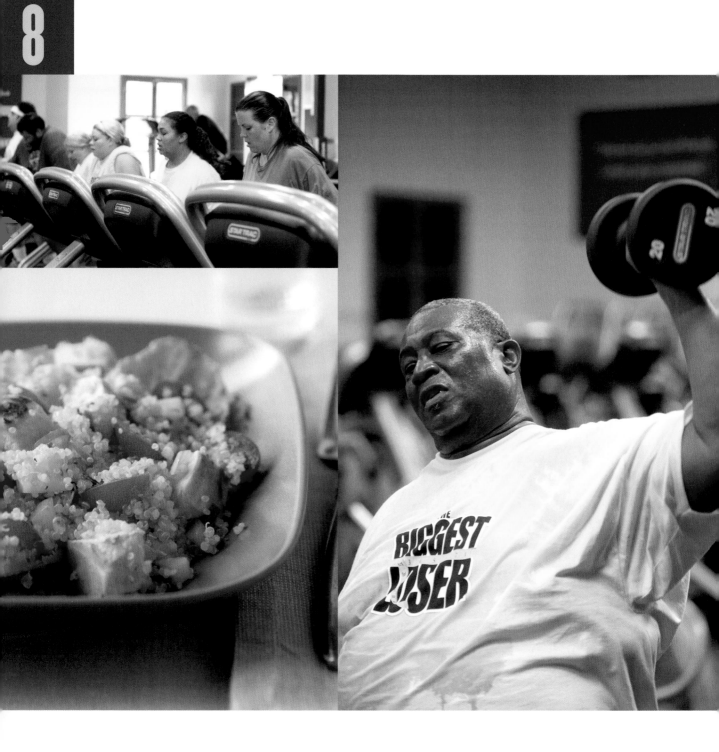

8

Week 5: Mind Your Health

Getting your body moving and feeding it with nutritious foods are two key components of weight loss—but at the end of the day, any serious commitment to weight loss and improved health is all in your head. Weight loss and maintenance are entirely dependent on a strong mental strategy and the ability to keep your head in the game.

Part of what makes *The Biggest Losers'* transformations so awe-inspiring is not just the dramatic physical change of dropping several pant or dress sizes: It's the clarity of mind and the renewed appetite for life that come with a healthier body.

It should come as no surprise that the effects of eating right and exercising do a number—and a good one—on your mind as much as your body.

Vicky Vilcan, the contestant everyone loved to hate in Season 6, describes the new mental outlook she has today: "When I was leaving the Ranch, I left Bob Harper a note telling him there was a small 'glass half full' spot in my heart that he had put there. I am happy to say that it has

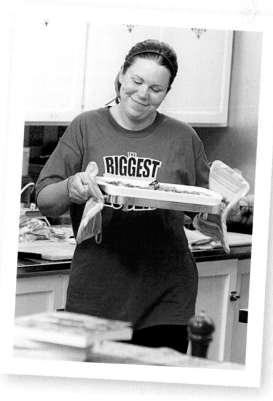

grown and taken over just about everything I do. When I go outside, I appreciate everything from the blue sky to the green grass. I love the culture and people of the community I live in. I am grateful to have made a new network of friends. It's weird when I think about it: I'm sitting here, eating fresh berries for lunch, thinking, "Thank you to the man who worked hard to farm these fresh, juicy berries just for me." I mean, really . . . did pessimistic Vicky just think that?! Yes, she did, and I truly love her."

New Dreams

After only a few weeks on the Ranch, the contestants notice that their attitudes start to shift and they feel better. Eleven years ago, Season 9 contestant Sherry Johnston was faced with the daunting

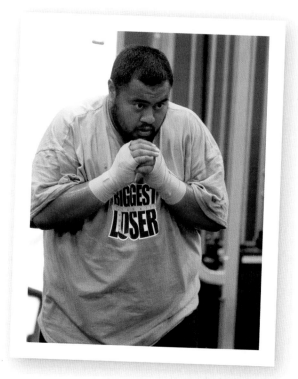

Tara Costa, Season 7 Finalist

I lead a new healthy lifestyle, a lifestyle I want to live. And I finally believe that I am worth it. I'm hoping that I can give that back to other people.

challenge of raising a family on her own after her husband died of cancer. She prioritized her children and her job first, and her own health came last. After she and daughter Ashley arrived on the Ranch, Sherry realized, "I want to change my life, my future! I am beginning to see a vision for *my* life. Instead of 'I can't do this' or 'I can't do that,' I'm gaining more of an 'I can' mentality as I feel better from eating healthy and exercising. I have a new drive and determination, and along with that come new dreams! I want to be that thin person I used to be, but this time I want to be *healthy*. I want to be a healthy mom for my children and grandchildren."

For Season 9 castmate Sam Poueu, losing more than 75 pounds in the course of about 2 months has helped him make peace with himself. "It's amazing how losing weight can help you feel more stable and centered," he says. "I feel better about myself than I ever have in my life. I am getting to know 'me,' and I have become well-rounded physically, mentally, and spiritually. When times are tough, I drink tea now instead of turning to alcohol. I'm high on life—I don't need anything else to get me going! Feeling good is an addiction!"

Even O'Neal Hampton, who had to return home for 30 days after losing a challenge on his first day at the Ranch with daughter SunShine, found that after 30 days of clean living and working out, he felt more positive and more driven. "My ideas are more my ideas. As you lose the weight, you can see who you truly are."

A Long, Good Life

These days people are living longer than ever. In the coming decades, the number of people who live to an advanced age will swell dramatically. While it's exciting to think that we have more years to enjoy, for some people, the prospect of living longer is overshadowed by the troubling possibility of eventual memory loss, dementia, and Alzheimer's disease.

Though occasional memory slips and "senior moments" are nothing to worry about, many of us (especially those of us who have witnessed the mental decline of our aging parents) worry that those lapses could signal the onset of Alzheimer's. People with this cruel and heartbreaking disease have trouble with simple tasks, struggle with words, forget faces and names, and get lost in familiar settings. They may behave inappropriately and show sudden mood swings. In later stages, people with Alzheimer's can no longer recognize their families or function independently.

Although experts still don't know exactly what causes Alzheimer's disease—and therefore aren't completely certain how to prevent it—the evidence

Alexandra White, Season 8

It's important to believe in yourself—because no one else can do it for you. You have to have the will and the drive to do it yourself. If you have those things, then you can lose the weight.

is accumulating that there are sensible steps you can take to keep your brain healthy and provide some protection from mental decline.

About Dementia and Alzheimer's

Your brain contains 100 billion nerve cells called neurons. These allow you to process information, store memories, communicate, and do the other things that you consider "thinking."

When any of a number of disorders interferes with the function of your neurons, dementia can result. Memory loss, a common symptom, in and of itself does not constitute dementia; instead, doctors diagnose dementia only if two or more brain functions—such as memory, language skills, perception, or cognitive skills, including reasoning and judgment—are significantly impaired.

Alzheimer's disease is the most common cause of dementia, accounting for 60 to 80 percent of cases and affecting 5.3 million Americans. After Alzheimer's, the second-most-common cause of dementia is what's known as vascular dementia, caused by brain damage from cerebrovascular or cardiovascular problems, most commonly in the form of a series of small strokes—blockages or ruptures in blood vessels feeding the brain. Vascular dementia accounts for up to 20 percent of all dementia.

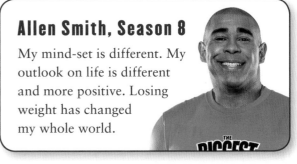

Allen Smith, Season 8

My mind-set is different. My outlook on life is different and more positive. Losing weight has changed my whole world.

Risk Factors

Age is the biggest risk factor for developing a condition that causes dementia. As you progress through your later years, the chance that you'll develop Alzheimer's will rise steeply. Fewer than 1 percent of people in their early 60s have the condition. After the age of 65, the number rises to 10 percent. And almost half of people over the age of 85 have Alzheimer's.

Because women live longer, on average, than men, women are more likely to develop Alzheimer's disease and other dementias. Family history is another risk factor. Research has shown that those who have a parent, brother or sister, or child with Alzheimer's are twice as likely to develop the disease as those without a family history.

Heart health is a key consideration in prevention. Because vascular dementia is caused by small strokes, which are in turn caused by damage to the blood vessels (as described in Chapter 5), those at risk for cardiovascular disease are also considered at risk for developing dementia.

Vascular (blood vessel) disease may also contribute to Alzheimer's, though experts still are unclear about the connection. A number of factors that raise your risk of heart disease are associated with a higher risk of Alzheimer's, including diabetes, high cholesterol, high blood pressure, and smoking. In addition, research has shown that a higher-than-average blood level of homocysteine—a type of amino acid—is a strong risk factor for the development of Alzheimer's and vascular dementia.

What to Watch For: Recognizing a Pattern

According to the Alzheimer's Association, you should seek guidance from your physician if you experience these symptoms:

- Memory loss that disrupts daily life
- Misplacing things without the ability to retrace steps
- Challenges in planning or solving problems
- Difficulty completing familiar tasks
- Ongoing confusion about time or place
- Trouble understanding visual images or spatial relationships
- New problems speaking or writing
- Decreased or poor judgment
- Withdrawal from work or social activities
- Changes in mood or personality

People with vascular dementia may exhibit similar symptoms, but the onset is likely to be more sudden, after one or several small strokes. When the disease does get worse, it often progresses in

Junk-Food Brain

Did you know that what you eat can affect your mood? Processed foods that contain refined sugar and carbohydrates are obviously terrible for your waistline—and they aren't doing your brain any favors, either. Processed "junk" foods cause your blood sugar to spike and then rapidly crash, resulting in fatigue, irritability, brain fog, and depression.

In fact, a recent study published in the *British Journal of Psychiatry* makes a strong case that processed junk food can trigger or contribute to depression, while eating whole foods seems to be protective. Scientists found that consumption of processed foods was associated with increased likelihood of depression, whereas those who had the highest consumption of whole foods were the least likely to be depressed.

steps, with sudden changes in ability. Unlike people with Alzheimer's, people with vascular dementia often maintain their personalities and normal levels of emotional responsiveness until the later stages of the disease.

It's important to note that an occasional, individual symptom on its own is normal. You've probably lost your keys from time to time—that's perfectly normal. When you're healthy, you find the keys by reviewing in your mind all the places you've recently been where you might have left them. But people with Alzheimer's can't solve the problem because their memory, judgment, and problem-solving faculties are impaired.

If you do suspect the onset of dementia, seek guidance from your health care provider, who can rule out an array of treatable conditions such as depression, drug interaction, thyroid problems, excessive use of alcohol, or certain vitamin deficiencies.

The Weight-Loss Connection

Just as the foods you eat work in concert to keep your body healthy, they also maintain your brain health. Your diet and lifestyle choices can help you prevent Alzheimer's disease and other mental deterioration as you age.

As mentioned, the amino acid homocysteine has been linked to the development of dementia and Alzheimer's disease. As homocysteine levels rise, so does the risk of these conditions. You can lower your levels of this substance by raising your levels of vitamins B_6, B_{12}, and folate (also known as folic acid). Doing so can help protect you from homocysteine's harmful effects. Use the recommendations that follow to keep your brain healthy and help prevent degenerative diseases.

Boost Your B Vitamins

Load up on folate-rich fruits and vegetables, such as:

- Bananas
- Beans and lentils
- Chickpeas and black-eyed peas
- Green leafy vegetables, such as Chinese cabbage,

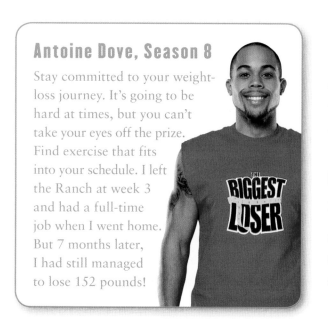

Antoine Dove, Season 8

Stay committed to your weight-loss journey. It's going to be hard at times, but you can't take your eyes off the prize. Find exercise that fits into your schedule. I left the Ranch at week 3 and had a full-time job when I went home. But 7 months later, I had still managed to lose 152 pounds!

collard greens, lettuce, mustard greens, spinach, and turnip greens

- Green peas
- Other vegetables, such as artichokes, asparagus, beets, broccoli, brussels sprouts, cauliflower, okra, potatoes, red bell peppers, and scallions
- Sunflower seeds

Many of the same foods supply vitamin B_6; for an additional B boost, incorporate these foods into your diet:

- Avocado
- Crude or unprocessed wheat bran
- Lean pork loin
- Skinless chicken breast
- Soybeans
- Walnuts

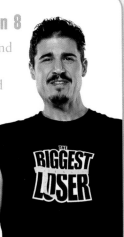

Julio Gomez, Season 8

I have changed by leaps and bounds since losing 180 pounds—body, mind, and soul. I'm stronger and healthier, physically and mentally. I am no longer afraid. Life will be different from this point forward, and I'm grateful for it.

SunShine Hampton, Season 9

Here's a visualization tool when workouts get tough: When lifting weights, push all the negative thoughts out through your hands. When you run on the treadmill, push all the negative thoughts out through your feet.

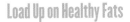

Load Up on Healthy Fats

The human brain is 60 percent fat. The vitamins A, B_{12}, D, and K are fat soluble. Your body cannot absorb these nutrients without fats—so it's important that you get enough healthy fats in your diet to promote optimal brain function.

Omega-3s are a type of polyunsaturated fatty acid. The chief omega-3 in the brain is DHA (docosahexaenoic acid), which is found in the fatty membranes that surround nerve cells, especially in the places where cells connect to one another. Eicosapentaenoic acid (EPA) is another type of omega-3 fatty acid and is required for the production of a special group of substances in the body called prostaglandins, which control blood clotting.

Research has linked certain types of omega-3s

to a reduced risk of heart disease and stroke—and a number of studies now suggest that omega-3s can also reduce the risk of dementia or cognitive decline. In addition, omega-3 deficiencies have been linked to depression.

When it comes to Alzheimer's, the latest research suggests that omega-3s can help reverse symptoms only if administered in the earliest stages, so incorporating them into your daily diet now is the best strategy for long-term brain health. At one time, omega-3s were abundant in our food supply. Now that we eat more processed and fast foods, most of us have become deficient in this important nutrient. To increase your intake:

- **Eat cold-water fish at least three times per week.** Fish are your best source of omega-3s and make a satisfying substitute for red meat. Just be sure to cook fish healthfully! The table on this page lists the varieties of fish that are richest in omega-3s.

Fish	EPA/DHA content
Pacific herring, baked (3½ oz)	1.2 g EPA/0.9 g DHA
Chinook salmon fillet, baked (3½ oz)	1.0 g EPA/0.7 g DHA
Anchovies (3½ oz)	0.8 g EPA/1.3 g DHA
Greenland halibut fillet (3½ oz)	0.7 g EPA/0.5 g DHA
Sockeye salmon (3½ oz)	0.5 g EPA/0.7 g DHA
Wild coho salmon (3½ oz)	0.5 g EPA/0.5 g DHA

- **Add flax.** Whole flaxseed, ground flaxseed, and flaxseed oil pack a hefty omega-3 punch. Use flaxseed oil to cook or in vinaigrette dressings; sprinkle whole or ground flaxseeds in yogurt or on breakfast cereal to get an omega-3 boost.

- **Don't forget the eggs.** In recent years, an improved source of omega-3s has been finding its way into supermarkets and onto dinner tables: the egg. You can now buy eggs containing extra omega-3s; they're produced by giving chickens a diet containing flaxseed. One large enriched egg contains about 225 milligrams of omega-3s, compared with 80 milligrams in a regular egg. They cost a bit more than regular eggs, but they're yet another source of a key antiaging nutrient that's too often scarce in our diets.

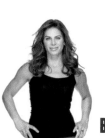

Biggest Loser Trainer Tip: Jillian Michaels

Let go of that whole identity of being a failure, of being less than, of not being able to do it, blah blah blah. Let go of the story. Until you're ready to step into a new life and write a new story, you're just wasting your time.

Keep Your Brain and Body Active

The effects of physical exercise on the brain should not be underestimated. A study published in the journal *Sports Medicine* found that exercise led to a significant drop in depressive symptoms. In addition, scientists at the University of Illinois at Urbana-Champaign studied a group of men and women between the ages of 55 and 79 and found that physically fit participants had less age-related brain-tissue shrinkage than less active subjects. But you don't need a scientific study to prove that exercising just plain makes you feel better, sharper, and more alert. As Season 7's Carla Triplett says, "I'm on the go without being exhausted. I no longer have to mask my feelings and pretend to be happy—I *am* happy!"

Mental exercises may also help to boost your brainpower by allowing the brain to develop and maintain connections between neurons. In other words, if you don't want to lose it, use it! Here are some easy mental exercises to keep your brain sharp.

- **Learn new things.** Check out library books about unfamiliar subjects. Watch educational TV programs that challenge you to think about new topics. Take classes at your local community center.
- **Tease your brain.** Do crosswords, sudoku, and other puzzles every day. Memorize short lists of objects—such as items on your shopping list. Bring up old memories or look through photo albums and try to remember details.
- **Call a friend.** A Swedish study from 2002 found that those who engaged in frequent social activities had roughly 40 percent less risk of developing dementia. So pick up the phone and stay connected!

Rudy Pauls, Season 8

Before I came to the Ranch, I wasn't a huge fish eater. But now I like halibut and tilapia, and my favorite is orange roughy with lemon-pepper seasoning and fresh mango salsa. I also love tacos with ground turkey sautéed in a nonstick skillet with onions and mushrooms. Get the low-carb tortillas. Add lettuce, tomato, and fat-free Greek-style yogurt as a substitute for sour cream.

Week 5 Menu Plan

MONDAY   1,430 calories

Breakfast

Jerry and Estella's Veggie Cheese Omelet
(page 72)

1 slice whole grain toast

1 cup cubed honeydew melon

1 cup fat-free milk

Snack

1 large apple

½ ounce walnuts

Lunch

Out-to-Lunch Tostada Salad (page 251)

1 cup fat-free tomato soup

1 cup fat-free milk

Snack

1 serving **Frozen Berry-Nut Parfait** (page 208)

Dinner

1 serving **Tortilla-Free Burrito** (page 211) with
3 slices (1 ounce) avocado

1 cup fresh berries and ½ banana, sliced

1 cup fat-free milk

Green tea or coffee

TUESDAY   1,582 calories

Breakfast

3 **Breakfast "Tacos"** (page 213)

½ cup fresh salsa

1 cup fat-free milk

½ cup cubed watermelon or other melon

Snack

1 stick low-fat Cheddar cheese

1 large apple

Lunch

1½ cups low-fat minestrone

1 cup baby spinach with 1 teaspoon low-fat
dressing and 1 tablespoon ground flaxseed

Iced green tea or black tea

Snack

My German Lover (page 256)

Dinner

1 serving **Ed and Heba's Blue-Ribbon Chicken**
(page 214)

1 artichoke, steamed

1 cup fat-free milk

WEDNESDAY   1,580 calories

Breakfast

¼ cup steel-cut oatmeal cooked with
1 tablespoon wheat bran and 1 cup
unsweetened vanilla almond milk

1 hard-boiled egg

1 large orange

Green tea or coffee

Snack

1 ounce smoked salmon

2 Wasa crackers

Lunch

Biggest Loser BLTE (page 246)

1 fresh pear

1 cup fat-free milk

Snack

1 cup steamed edamame

Dinner

5 ounces wild salmon, grilled

1 cup brussels sprouts roasted with 1 teaspoon
olive oil

¾ cup cooked wild rice

THURSDAY   1,550 calories

Breakfast

1 cup Kashi GoLean cereal and 1 tablespoon
ground flaxseed

1 cup unsweetened vanilla almond milk

¾ cup fresh blueberries

¾ cup fat-free vanilla yogurt

Snack

½ tuna salad sandwich on whole grain bread

1 cup fat-free milk

Lunch

1 serving **Quinoa Tabbouleh with Roast Turkey
and Tomatoes** (page 217)

1 cup green grapes

Iced tea

Snack

½ cup fat-free cottage cheese with ½ cup fresh
salsa

Dinner

1 serving **Moussaka** (page 218)

2 cups mixed greens with 3 slices avocado;
6 cherry tomatoes, halved; and 1 tablespoon
low-fat vinaigrette

Green tea

FRIDAY
1,480 calories

Breakfast

Patti's Melt (page 105)

1 banana, sliced, with ½ cup fresh raspberries

Green tea or coffee

Snack

2 hard-boiled eggs, yolks scooped out, stuffed with 4 tablespoons hummus

Lunch

Shrimp cocktail: 8 boiled or grilled large shrimp with ¼ cup spicy cocktail sauce

2 cups **Fire-Roasted Tomato Soup** (page 252)

1 cup fat-free milk

Snack

1½ cups steamed edamame

Dinner

6 ounces halibut baked with lemon and low-sodium seasoning

1 small baked sweet potato

1 cup steamed broccoli

Green tea or coffee

SATURDAY
1,530 calories

Breakfast

French toast: 1 slice whole grain bread and 1 omega-3-enriched egg

1 tablespoon sugar-free fruit spread

3 slices turkey bacon

½ large red grapefruit

Coffee

Snack

2 slices low-fat provolone cheese and 2 slices lean roast turkey on 4 whole grain crackers (or 2 Wasa crackers)

Lunch

1½ cups low-fat split-pea soup with 1 ounce chopped Canadian bacon

1 pear

1 cup fat-free milk

Snack

2 **Andrea's Roast Beef Roll-Ups** (page 81)

Dinner

6 ounces filet mignon, grilled

¾ cup cooked whole grain pasta with 1 tablespoon pesto

2 Roma tomatoes, sliced, with 1 tablespoon balsamic vinegar

Green tea or coffee

SUNDAY   1,435 calories

Breakfast

Sunrise Shake (page 221) with 1 tablespoon
  ground flaxseed

1 low-fat bran muffin

1 cup fat-free milk

Coffee or green tea

Snack

2 ounces lean deli ham

1 large wedge cantaloupe or honeydew melon

Lunch

1 **Mexican Turkey Burger** (page 82) on whole
  grain bun

½ cup salsa and ¼ medium avocado

Iced tea

Snack

¾ cup fat-free ricotta cheese, ½ cup cherries
  (or blackberries), and 1 tablespoon toasted
  slivered almonds

Dinner

1 serving **Moroccan Pork Stew with Baby
  Artichokes and Dried Fruit** (page 112)

¾ cup cooked whole wheat couscous

2 plums or apricots

Green tea

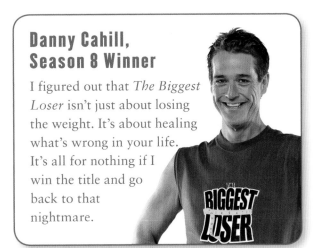

Danny Cahill, Season 8 Winner

I figured out that *The Biggest Loser* isn't just about losing the weight. It's about healing what's wrong in your life. It's all for nothing if I win the title and go back to that nightmare.

FROZEN BERRY-NUT PARFAIT

If Season 9 contestant Michael Ventrella's not in the gym, you can usually find him in the Ranch kitchen, inventing a new and delicious concoction. This is a special dessert he created one night for his mother and teammate, Maria.

1	cup plain, fat-free Greek-style yogurt
½	cup fresh blueberries
⅓	cup diced frozen strawberries
1–2	packets Truvia or other natural sweetener
2	teaspoons vanilla extract
¼	cup chopped walnuts, toasted

In a food processor, combine the yogurt, blueberries, strawberries, sweetener, and vanilla and process until smooth. Stir in the nuts. Transfer the mixture to a pint container, cover, and freeze for about 30 minutes, or until just frozen. Scoop into 4 parfait glasses and serve immediately.

Note: This dessert can be served later, but it will form ice crystals if frozen longer than directed and thus won't be as creamy.

Note: If you opt to leave out the nuts, the calories are halved, or 45 per serving.

Makes 4 (½-cup) servings

Per serving: 90 calories, 7 g protein, 6 g carbohydrates (4 g sugars), 4 g fat (0 g saturated), 0 mg cholesterol, 1 g fiber, 20 mg sodium

Mo DeWalt, Season 8

At 355 pounds, I think I had forgotten who I was. Now, at 263 pounds, I have found some strong resolve and knowledge. Let changes come into your life—don't allow yourself to go back to that person you used to be.

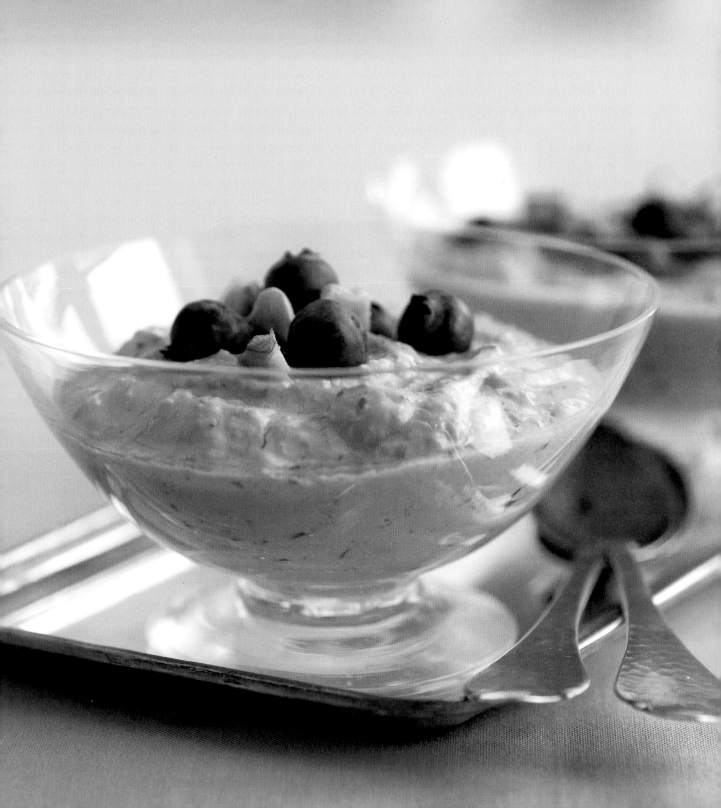

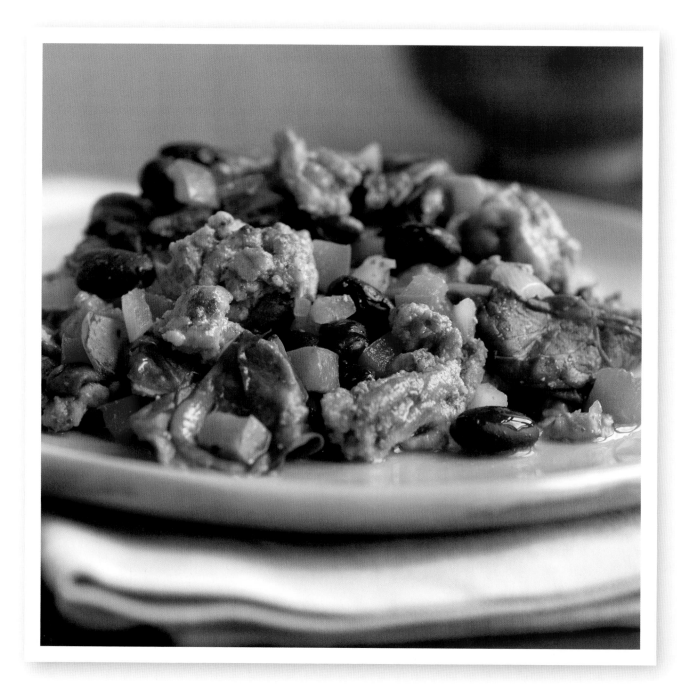

TORTILLA-FREE BURRITO

This high-protein dish is a staple in Season 4 contestant Nicole Michalik's kitchen. "I try not to eat carbs after 5:00 p.m., so I make this for dinner. It's perfect with salsa and guacamole. I don't even miss the tortilla," she says. This recipe makes about 8 cups, so it's easy to freeze some for later.

1¼ **pounds lean ground turkey**

1 **medium yellow onion, chopped**

1 **cup diced yellow, red, or green bell pepper (about 1 medium pepper)**

1 **tablespoon chili powder**

1 **teaspoon ground cumin**

1 **teaspoon ground mustard**

1 **teaspoon oregano**

Red chile flakes (optional)

1½ **cups cooked black or kidney beans, or 1 (15-ounce) can, rinsed and drained**

1 **(10-ounce) package frozen spinach, thawed, or 10 cups fresh baby spinach**

Cilantro

Coat a large nonstick skillet or Dutch oven with cooking spray. Add the turkey, onion, and bell pepper and simmer for about 5 minutes, until just cooked through.

Add the chili powder, cumin, mustard, oregano, and chile flakes, if desired. Stir well. Add the beans and spinach and cook just until heated through. Season to taste. Garnish with cilantro.

Makes 8 (1-cup) servings

Per serving: 140 calories, 21 g protein, 12 g carbohydrates (1 g sugars), 2 g fat (0 g saturated), 30 mg cholesterol, 5 g fiber, 105 mg sodium

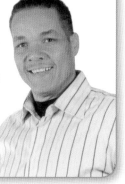

Pete Thomas, Season 2

Some foods we like because of the texture in our mouths. For example, I use really lean hamburger, but it dries out easily. So I take a bit of unflavored gelatin and mix it in with the burger to add a little moisture and make the meat taste more succulent. It takes the place of adding an egg to the beef.

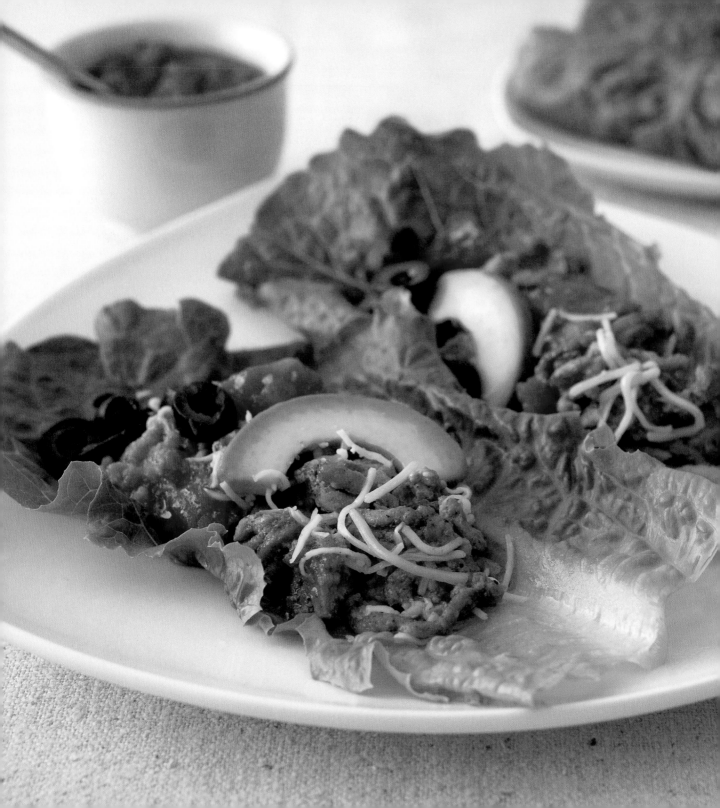

BREAKFAST "TACOS"

This delicious, portable meal slashes the carbs and ramps up the protein. It can be eaten any time of day and is a perfect postworkout snack or meal to take on the go. Mix up the filling for these taco-style wraps and store in the fridge. Wrap in lettuce and you're ready to go!

3   large romaine lettuce leaves

4   ounces cooked 99% fat-free ground turkey seasoned with ½ teaspoon low-sodium taco seasoning

½   cup fat-free refried beans

¼   cup reduced-fat Mexican four-cheese blend

2   tablespoons sliced black olives

2   tablespoons fresh tomato salsa

3   slices avocado (optional)

Using the lettuce leaves as taco shells, place ⅓ of the turkey, beans, cheese, olives, and salsa on one end of each leaf. Add an avocado slice, if desired, and roll each leaf like a wrap, tucking in the edges.

Makes 3 (1-taco) servings

Per serving: **150 calories, 17 g protein, 11 g carbohydrates (0 g sugars), 5 g fat (2 g saturated), 25 mg cholesterol, 4 g fiber, 310 mg sodium**

Amanda Arlauskas, Season 8 Finalist

I was so sad when I began this journey at 250 pounds. But what finally changed was my mind-set. If you keep telling yourself you're going to fail, you'll fail. It just clicked for me. I realized that I *could* run on the treadmill and I could run a lot longer than I thought possible.

ED AND HEBA'S BLUE-RIBBON CHICKEN

One night when Season 6 finalist Heba Salama was craving something Italian and her husband, Ed Brantley, was in the mood for the flavor of rosemary, they put their heads together and came up with this tasty dish. They already had all the ingredients in the refrigerator, and you probably do, too!

2 tablespoons Dijon mustard

4 (4-ounce) boneless, skinless chicken breasts, trimmed of fat and butterflied

4 slices low-sodium ham

4 slices 2% Swiss or low-fat provolone cheese

Salt and ground black pepper to taste

1 teaspoon fresh rosemary, chopped

¼ cup fat-free, low-sodium chicken broth

Spread the mustard evenly inside the 4 chicken breasts. In a small non-stick skillet over medium heat, quickly sear the ham for about 30 seconds on each side. Place a slice of ham on 1 side of each piece of chicken. Place 1 slice of cheese folded in half over the top of the ham. Fold over the butterflied chicken breast to create a pocket. Tuck in the cheese so it's well concealed. Season each breast with salt, pepper, and rosemary.

Lightly coat a skillet with cooking oil spray. Gently place each breast in the pan. Cook on medium to low heat for 6 to 8 minutes, until golden brown, then turn over the breasts and brown the other side. Once the chicken is fully cooked, remove it from the pan momentarily and drain any excess grease from the skillet. Return the skillet to the heat, add the broth, then place the chicken in the broth. Simmer for 3 to 4 minutes. Serve immediately.

Makes 4 servings

Per serving: 220 calories, 37 g protein, 2 g carbohydrates (0 g sugars), 7 g fat (3 g saturated), 85 mg cholesterol, 0 g fiber, 460 mg sodium

Ashley Johnston, Season 9

What motivates me to keep going when it gets tough is seeing the progress I've already made and how different I look and feel. I want to keep going so I feel even better and am able to do more. Just starting to feel beautiful again motivates me to keep burning those calories and seeing those results. I want to start my life over. That's what motivates me to get up and do this day after day!

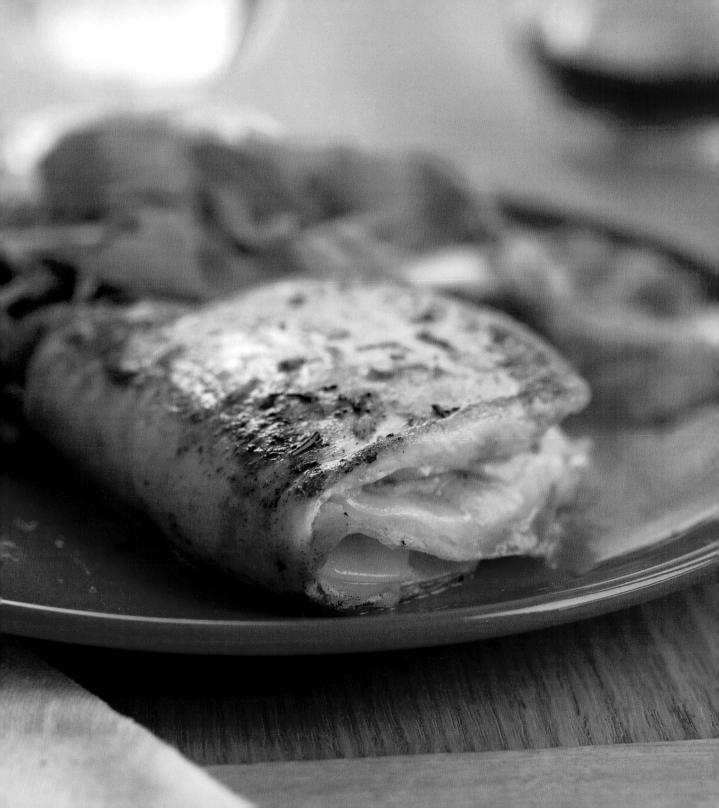

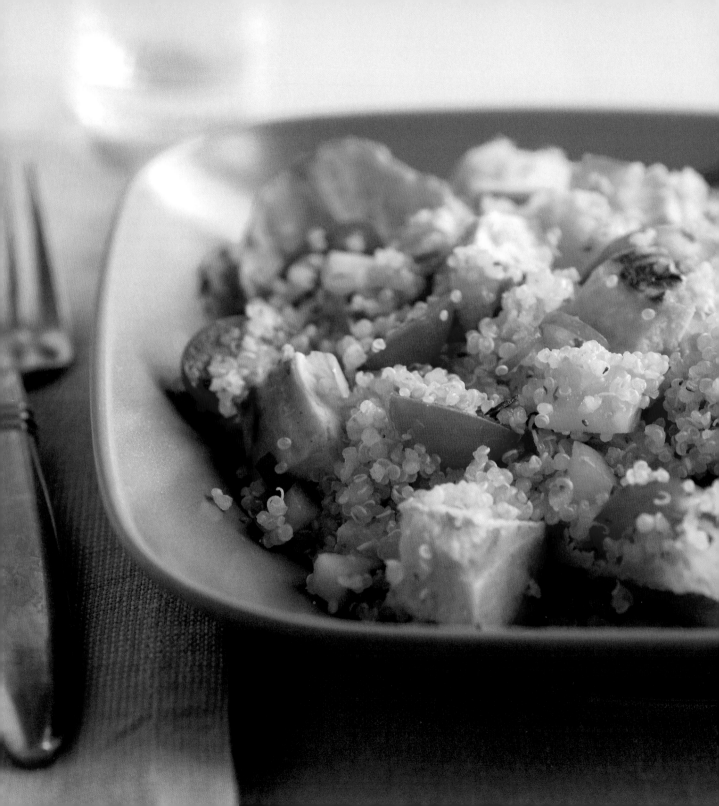

QUINOA TABBOULEH WITH ROAST TURKEY AND TOMATOES

Like the conventional tabbouleh, this version made with quinoa contains more veggies than grains. Quinoa is thought of as a whole grain, but technically it's a high-protein seed native to South America. You can eat this as a salad, wrap a serving in lettuce leaves, tuck a serving in a whole wheat pita, or serve it as a side dish.

2 cups water

1 cup dry quinoa

2 cups halved cherry tomatoes (or 2 tomatoes, seeded and diced)

1 cup diced, seeded, peeled cucumber

¼ cup chopped fresh Italian parsley

¼ cup lemon juice

1 tablespoon extra-virgin olive oil

1 tablespoon grated lemon peel

¾ teaspoon salt

¼ teaspoon ground black pepper

2 scallions (white and green parts), finely chopped

2 cups shredded or diced roast turkey breast (without skin)

Place the water and quinoa in a 1-quart saucepan. Bring to a boil, cover, and turn down the heat to a low simmer. Let the quinoa cook for about 15 minutes, then remove the pan from the heat and allow the grain to cool.

Meanwhile, in a medium mixing bowl, combine the tomatoes, cucumber, parsley, lemon juice, oil, lemon peel, salt, pepper, and all but 1 tablespoon of the scallions. Add the cooled quinoa to the mixture and stir just to blend. Cover and chill.

To serve, divide the tabbouleh among 4 plates. Top with the turkey. Garnish with the reserved scallion. This dish can be made 1 day in advance.

Makes 4 (1¼-cup) servings

Per serving: 310 calories, 27 g protein, 35 g carbohydrates (3 g sugars), 7 g fat (1 g saturated), 35 mg cholesterol, 3 g fiber, 420 mg sodium

Daniel Wright, Season 8

A new healthy food I found at the Ranch was quinoa—it's like a healthy brown rice, but it also has protein. I spray just a tiny bit of butter substitute on it.

MOUSSAKA

This classic meat and eggplant dish is typically made with lamb. Here, lean ground turkey is simmered in richly seasoned tomatoes and chunks of sun-dried tomatoes. Allowing the flavors to meld intensifies the flavor: This moussaka is even more delicious the day after it's been baked, and it freezes well for up to a month.

Meat Mixture

- 2 teaspoons olive oil
- 1¼ pounds lean ground turkey
- 1 cup chopped yellow onion
- ¾ cup white wine or fat-free chicken or vegetable broth
- 1¾ cups (15 ounces) low-sodium tomato sauce
- 1 tablespoon chopped fresh oregano or 1 teaspoon dried
- 1 teaspoon ground nutmeg
- 1 teaspoon ground cinnamon
- 1 tablespoon honey

Béchamel Sauce

- 3 tablespoons canola or olive oil
- ¼ cup white whole wheat flour
- ¼ teaspoon ground black pepper
- 1 tablespoon minced garlic
- 1½ cups 1% milk
- ¾ cup fat-free chicken or vegetable broth
- ½ cup chopped scallions (white and green parts)
- ¾ cup finely chopped sun-dried tomatoes
- Salt and ground black pepper to taste
- 1 medium eggplant (about 1¼ pounds), washed, halved lengthwise, and sliced crosswise into ¼"-thick rounds
- ⅓ cup grated Parmesan cheese

To make the meat mixture: In a large, heavy saucepan, heat the oil over medium-high heat. Add the turkey and onion. Cook, stirring to break up the turkey, for about 5 minutes, until the meat is no longer pink. Add the wine or broth, tomato sauce, oregano, nutmeg, cinnamon, and honey. Simmer, stirring occasionally, for about 30 minutes, until the mixture thickens and is almost dry.

To make the béchamel sauce: In a 2-quart saucepan over medium heat, heat the oil. Whisk in the flour and pepper. Cook for 1 to 2 minutes, stirring constantly with a whisk. Add the garlic and cook until softened; do not brown. Pour in the milk and broth all at once. Cook over low heat, stirring constantly, until thickened and bubbly. Remove from the heat; stir in the scallions and sun-dried tomatoes. Season with salt and pepper. Set aside.

To assemble: Preheat the oven to 350°F. Lightly coat a 13" × 9" glass baking dish with cooking oil spray. Arrange half of the eggplant in the bottom of the dish. Add the meat mixture and spread in an even layer. Top with the remaining eggplant. Press down lightly with the palm of your hand to distribute evenly. Season with salt and pepper, if desired. Pour the hot béchamel sauce over the eggplant. Sprinkle with the cheese. Bake for about 1 hour, or until golden and bubbling on the edges. Cool for 10 minutes before serving.

Makes 8 (4½" x 3¼") servings

Per serving: 270 calories, 23 g protein, 23 g carbohydrates (9 g sugars), 9 g fat (2 g saturated), 35 mg cholesterol, 5 g fiber, 290 mg sodium

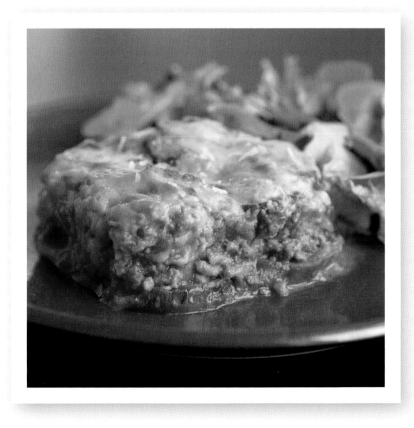

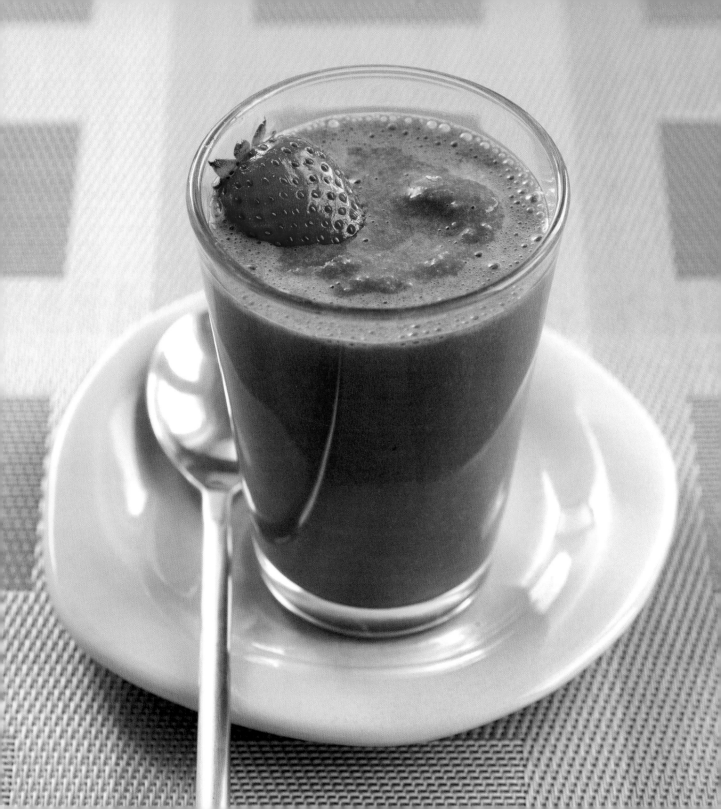

SUNRISE SHAKE

Like many other contestants, Season 9's Stephanie Anderson has a major sweet tooth. Though she likes this shake for breakfast, it's a great recovery drink after a workout, too, since it contains 7 grams of protein to help rebuild tired muscles.

1 cup Almond Breeze unsweetened vanilla almond milk

½ banana

½ cup sliced strawberries, frozen or fresh

2 scoops (4 tablespoons) *The Biggest Loser* chocolate protein powder

1 tablespoon unsweetened cocoa powder

1 teaspoon vanilla extract

1 package Truvia or other natural sweetener

1 cup ice

Combine the almond milk, banana, strawberries, protein powder, cocoa powder, vanilla, sweetener, and ice in a blender. Blend or puree until smooth. Pour into glasses and serve immediately.

Makes 2 (1½-cup) servings

Per serving: 100 calories, 7 g protein, 19 g carbohydrates (8 g sugars), 2 g fat (0 g saturated), 0 mg cholesterol, 8 g fiber, 85 mg sodium

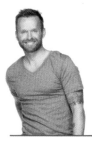

Biggest Loser Trainer Tip: Bob Harper

Make sure that after your workout, you give your body protein. You have to build the muscles back up because you've broken them down.

Week 5 Exercises

As we've seen, exercising your brain may help it develop and maintain connections between neurons that are important for protecting your mental faculties as you age. Those same neurons connect with skeletal muscles at a particular framework called the neuromuscular junction. There is a deep connection between mind and body, brain and muscle, and this connection actually stimulates brain cells to grow and connect. Staying active will not only keep your body healthy, it may also improve your brain function.

Any type of aerobic exercise (see Chapter 5) is great for a brain boost, because the heart-pumping action increases circulation and delivers oxygenated blood to the brain. Studies have shown that walking improves memory, focus, and the ability to learn, and can cut the risk of having a stroke in half! The good news is that *any* physical activity, even light-to-moderate or recreational activities, can improve brain function—but the more movement the better.

This week we are going to explore the mind-body connection through yoga. When people mention the term *yoga*, they usually refer to hatha yoga, the most popular branch of yoga, from which many styles originated, including power yoga, Bikram yoga, ashtanga yoga, and kundalini yoga. Most yoga styles use physical poses (known as *asanas*), breathing techniques (known as *pranayama*), and meditation to connect the mind and the body. Yoga develops physical strength and endurance, enhances functional flexibility, improves balance, and requires attention to detail, breath, and concentration. Just what you need to keep your brain turned on!

Focus: Yoga
Workout Guidelines

- Yoga is an ancient and complex practice. To get you started, in this workout we'll introduce a few key poses—all put together to form the Sun Salutation.

- Begin seated on a mat or carpeted surface with your legs crossed and your hands resting on your knees. Spend a few moments to center your mind. Simply focus on your breathing, taking notice of your body and how it feels, to prepare mentally and physically for the poses that follow. The Sun Salutation is often used as a warmup for more-rigorous yoga practices, so take your time and let your body guide you.

- Remember to breathe throughout the entire workout. Preferably breathe in and out through your nose. Fill your belly as you inhale, then exhale all the air out.

- Focus on correct alignment. Go only as far as you can while continuing to breathe freely. Holding your breath is a sign that you are pushing too far.

- Start with one circuit, or flow, of each pose and progress to 5 to 10 repetitions. Add 2 to 3 flows to any of the previous workouts as an active warmup or mobility cooldown. Or once you have built up to 10 or more flows, work in this yoga session to your full program as a restorative workout day. For example, try the cardio workout 3 days a week, strength/resistance and/or circuit workout 2 to 3 days a week, and finish up the week with the yoga flow.

- As always, consult your doctor before embarking on a new yoga routine. People with certain medical conditions may need to pay special attention to certain poses: Be cautious about forward and back bends if you have spine issues or are pregnant; extending your arms overhead if you have high blood pressure; and inversions if you have a neck injury, high blood pressure, or glaucoma.

Amanda Harmer, Season 5

Since getting healthy, I've gained the ability to spend good time with my family, be a better mommy and wife, get through my crazy daily routine without being exhausted, and hopefully live a longer, healthier life. I can appreciate how lucky I am to have so many wonderful opportunities. I'm learning that I always deserved all of these good things in my life, and I can't wait to see what's ahead!

SUN SALUTATION

The Sun Salutation gets the body moving through flexion and extension. It challenges both the upper and the lower body. Each pose can be performed independently and held for a few breaths or performed as a series, or flow. Start with one flow and progress to 5 to 10 repetitions. The Sun Salutation is a full cycle that includes:

1. Mountain Pose
2. Standing Forward Bend
3. Active Back Extension
4. Standing Forward Bend
5. Plank to Chaturanga
6. Upward-Facing Dog
7. Downward-Facing Dog
8. Standing Forward Bend
9. Mountain Pose

MOUNTAIN POSE

Stand with your feet together and your weight distributed evenly on both feet. "Lift" your kneecaps (keep your legs engaged) and "lift" your pelvis up and off your thighs. Keep your spine neutral, collarbones wide, chest open, and lower ribs softening in. Roll your shoulders down and back and place your arms by your sides, palms facing in. Keep your head, chin, and eyes level as you press the top of your skull toward the ceiling.

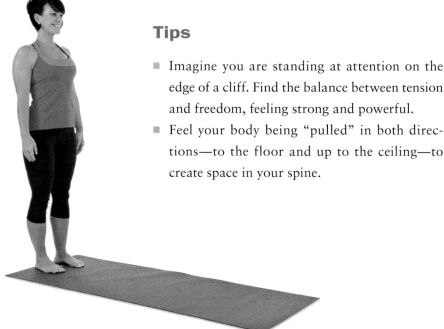

Tips

- Imagine you are standing at attention on the edge of a cliff. Find the balance between tension and freedom, feeling strong and powerful.
- Feel your body being "pulled" in both directions—to the floor and up to the ceiling—to create space in your spine.

STANDING FORWARD BEND

From Mountain Pose, inhale and extend your arms overhead, then exhale and sweep your arms as you hinge your torso down from your hips. Place your hands on the floor near your feet. Lift your buttocks up and off your thighs. Bring your chest close to your legs and relax your head and neck.

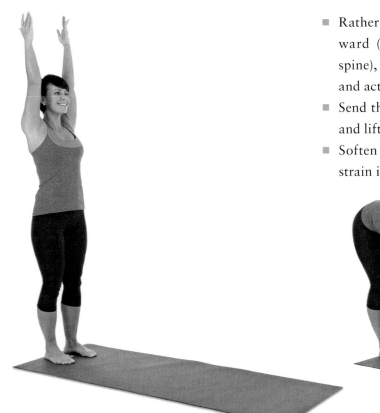

Tips

- Rather than completely release and relax forward (which can cause compression in the spine), draw your navel in toward your spine and actively move your chest to your thighs.
- Send the crown of your head toward your feet and lift your tailbone to the ceiling.
- Soften your knees (slightly bend) if you feel strain in the back of your knees, back, or neck.

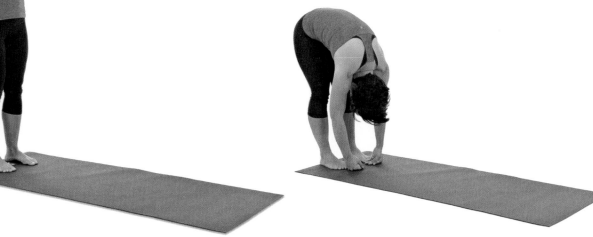

Beginner Modification

Place your hands on your shins or bend your knees.

Advanced Progression

As you reach overhead with your arms, extend your spine upward and lift your chest toward the ceiling.

ACTIVE BACK EXTENSION

From Standing Forward Bend, lift slightly to come to your fingertips, extend your spine, and look forward without crunching your neck (cervical spine). Release down to Standing Forward Bend.

Tips

- Pull your shoulder blades together to open your chest, but keep your neck long.
- Create length: Imagine tilting your tailbone to the ceiling at the same time you are drawing your navel toward your spine.
- Soften your knees (slightly bend) if you feel strain in the back of your knees or in your back or neck.

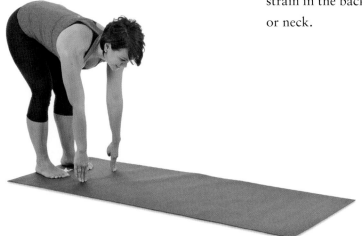

Beginner Modification

Place your hands on your shins.

Advanced Progression

Keep your palms flat on the floor.

PLANK TO CHATURANGA

The Plank is a transitional position before Chaturanga (lowering the body slowly toward the floor) that is also used for core stabilization. From Standing Forward Bend, step back with one leg and then the other, keeping your hands under your shoulders. Straighten your legs and keep your torso long so your body forms a straight line from head to heels. Maintain a neutral spine and draw your navel in. Move your shoulders away from your ears as you press into the floor. Keeping your elbows tight by your sides, slowly lower yourself to the floor, stopping as your arms come parallel to the floor.

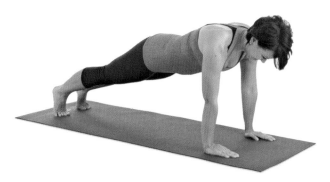

Tips

- Keep your legs active by reaching your heels behind you and by keeping your legs muscularly engaged and straight.
- Spread your fingers and press your hands into the floor.
- Don't allow your back to arch or your hips to dip when you lower yourself to the floor.

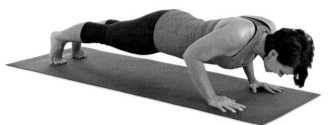

Beginner Modification
Place your knees on the floor.

Advanced Progression
Lift one leg as you lower yourself toward the floor. You may also jump both feet into Plank instead of stepping back into Plank.

UPWARD-FACING DOG

From Chaturanga, lead with your sternum, then raise your head and chest, straighten your arms, and lift your waist, hips, and thighs off the floor as you press into the tops of your feet. Bring your pelvis forward and keep your abdominals engaged. Stretch the front of your body without collapsing into your lower back or shoulders.

Tips

- Roll your shoulders down and back and open the front of your chest as you widen your collarbone.
- Keep your fingers spread on the floor, with your palms open and your middle fingers pointing forward.
- Lengthen your tailbone toward your feet and press your toenails down to the floor.

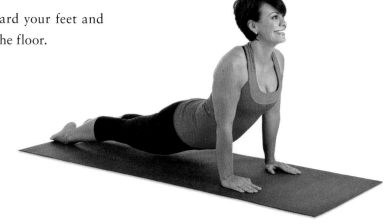

Beginner Modification

Keep your thighs on the floor or bend your elbows slightly. The goal is back extension—you don't want to let your shoulders creep up to your ears.

Advanced Progression

Look up and back, but be sure to support your neck on top of your shoulders. Don't let your neck release or drop.

DOWNWARD-FACING DOG

From Upward-Facing Dog, straighten your legs and arms and lift your hips and tailbone toward the ceiling. Your torso and head will hang between your arms so your body forms an inverted V. Reach your heels to the floor as you press your hands into the floor. Move your shoulders down away from your ears.

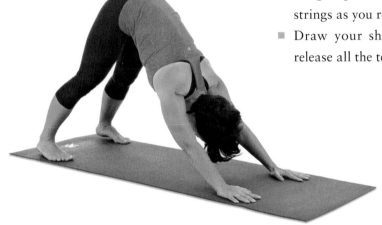

Tips

- Keep your fingers spread, with your palms open and your middle fingers pointing forward.
- Draw the muscles of your arms "up" into your shoulders.
- Imagine pressing your thighs back to your hamstrings as you reach your heels to the floor.
- Draw your shoulders down your back and release all the tension in your neck.

Beginner Modification
Keep your knees slightly bent. You may also come to your hands and knees between the Upward-Facing Dog and Downward-Facing Dog poses.

Advanced Progression
Extend one leg up toward the ceiling.

STANDING FORWARD BEND

From Downward-Facing Dog, step toward your hands and return to Standing Forward Bend (page 225). The advanced progression is to jump forward with your feet rather than step forward.

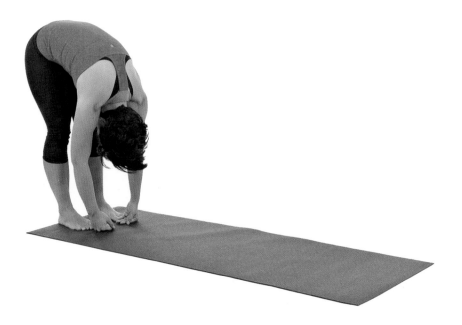

MOUNTAIN POSE

From Standing Forward Bend, sweep your arms out to the sides, lift your torso, and return to Mountain Pose (see page 224). Take a deep breath and settle into the pose.

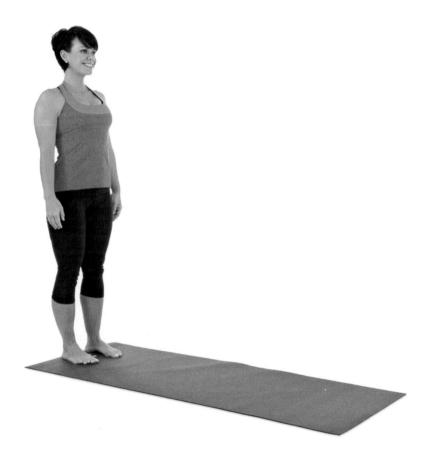

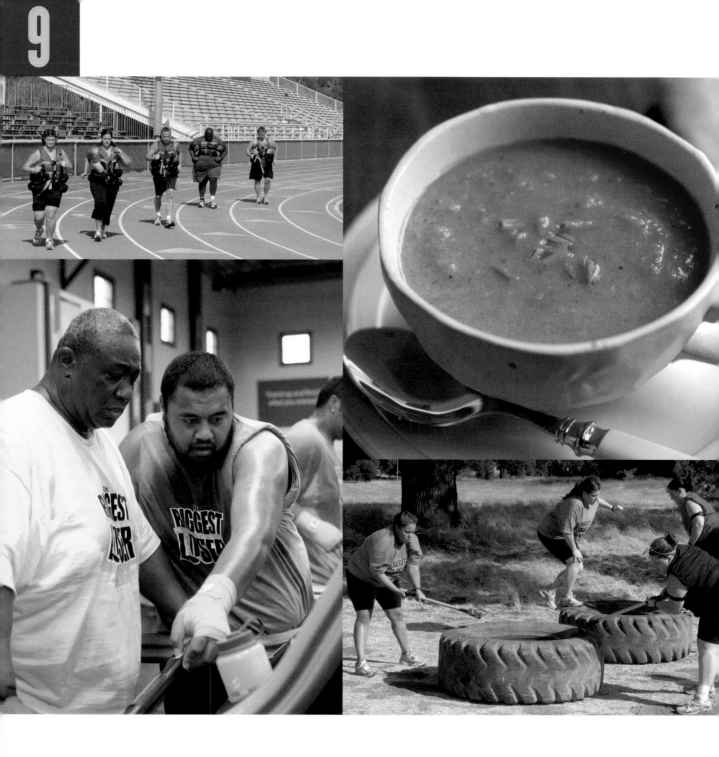

9

Week 6: Raise Your Defenses

We've all experienced the symptoms: fatigue, achiness, chills, and fever. When your body begins to feel run down, a more severe illness may be on the way. While you might want to crawl under a blanket and curse your weak immune system, you can actually take steps to protect yourself from getting sicker. And believe it or not, the symptoms above indicate that your immune system is already hard at work.

Nicole Michalik of Season 4 confesses that she has become "obsessed" with making sure that the majority of the foods she buys are organic and all natural. She also makes sure she eats tons of fruit and veggies. "I'm a stickler for having blueberries at least five times a week, as well as almonds, spinach, broccoli, and peppers," she says. "I honestly can see a huge difference in my health, especially in how few colds I get, just by making sure I am not only eating foods low in calories but also choosing good, healthy foods. Having more energy and seeing the benefits make you want to *keep* doing it.

"My friends call me the label police," laughs Nicole. "I refuse to buy (and rarely eat) *anything* with high-fructose corn syrup or partially hydrogenated oil. I am a firm believer in 'cleaner,' less-processed foods. The fewer ingredients, the better."

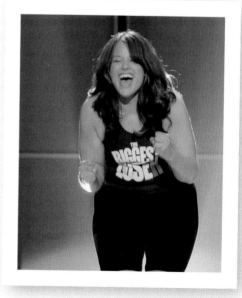

With all that good eating, she rarely gets the midafternoon slump. She is fueled and ready to get up at 6:45 every morning for work. After work, she hits the gym, then relaxes in front of the TV before heading off to bed.

Season 7's Sione Fa says he used to get headaches almost every day. He now realizes that his 12-can-a-day soda habit had something to do with that. "I used to come home at night and just drink soda the rest of the evening," he said. "After my second day on the Ranch and no soda, I noticed my headaches were gone. I haven't had one in a year." Season 7 castmate Estella Hayes says that she no longer suffers from debilitating sinus headaches, which she used to get frequently when she

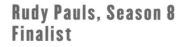

Rudy Pauls, Season 8 Finalist

Don't treat yourself to something "good" because you're having a bad day. Resolve to eat nutritious foods no matter what the situation. Sweat it out at the gym. It'll help you think through some of the problems you've been having.

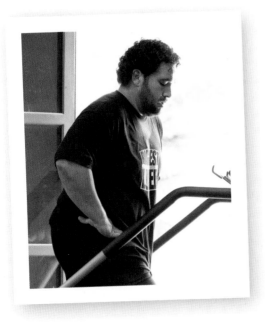

was eating unhealthy foods and not getting enough exercise.

"I feel much healthier today than I did before the show," says Vicky Vilcan of Season 6. "I have so much more energy and a more positive outlook on life. I remember feeling guilty because I was tired all the time and I could barely manage to keep up with working all day, the kids, and the housework. I felt like I was just existing and life was passing me by. Now I wake up at 4:30 every morning and run," says Vicky, who is training for a marathon. "I definitely lose an hour of sleep, but I get it back threefold in my energy and outlook for the remainder of the day."

And Kelly MacFarland from way-long-ago

Season 1 continues to be careful when choosing the food she eats. "Diabetes and heart disease are in my family, and I want to be sure that I don't add myself to the list. I try to eat a lot of fruits and veggies. Whole foods. Anything that will keep my body movin' and goovin' the way it's supposed to."

Kelly stays vigilant in keeping herself informed about health and fitness, always reading about the latest studies. "There are so many things that are different today," she says. "I rarely get sick. I sleep better. I used to sleep about 4 hours a night. I couldn't shut down enough to sleep. My body ached. Now I work out and eat healthy, so when bedtime comes, I'm ready. I used to take medicine for acid reflux and heartburn, but I haven't taken those meds since the day I stepped on the Ranch. I look forward to challenges and new things. It's exciting to feel good and do things I haven't done before."

About Your Immune System

The immune system is a complex network of your body's organs and tissues, which produce an array of cells that, in turn, create hormones and other substances. These carry information throughout the body, identify potentially harmful invaders, and serve as an elegant defense system to fight such invaders. Some of the important cells in the immune system include lymphocytes (white blood cells, including B and T cells), phagocytes (white blood cells that "eat" invaders), and cytokines (proteins).

In a streamlined process, this network of cells recognizes legitimate threats, coordinates the appropriate response, attacks invaders that can make you sick, and cleans up afterward. But sometimes this coordinated interaction breaks down or even backfires.

Some immune deficiency disorders arise when

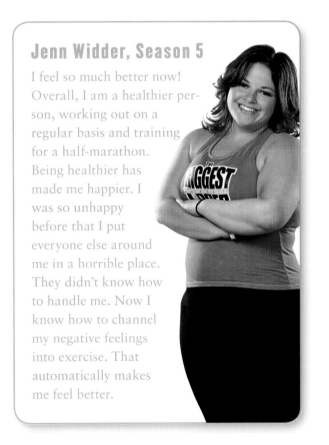

Jenn Widder, Season 5

I feel so much better now! Overall, I am a healthier person, working out on a regular basis and training for a half-marathon. Being healthier has made me happier. I was so unhappy before that I put everyone else around me in a horrible place. They didn't know how to handle me. Now I know how to channel my negative feelings into exercise. That automatically makes me feel better.

your immune system is missing one or more parts. This state can be debilitating in the long term, but most of us are more familiar with temporary immune deficiency, which may strike after you've been sick with a virus such as the flu or mononucleosis. Immune deficiency can also arise when new strains of viruses develop and your immune system fails to recognize and combat the new enemies fast enough—which is why the H1N1 virus, or swine flu—which caused nearly 5,000 hospitalizations in 6 weeks in the fall of 2009 and has claimed more than 10,000 lives in the United States—poses a threat to public health.

Autoimmune diseases arise when your immune system confuses your body's own cells with harmful outsiders and attacks them. Sometimes the damage is subtle; at other times it is progressive and deadly. More than 80 kinds of autoimmune diseases can develop, including rheumatoid arthritis and lupus, each of which affect more than 1.3 million Americans.

Inflammation is often a helpful reaction. When your body needs to heal a wound or protect you from an onslaught of germs entering via your bloodstream, it sends a swarm of cells to the affected area, causing heat and swelling. But ongoing inflammation may result in damage to your body, including increased production of free radicals, which further fuels the inflammatory fire in a vicious cycle. Inflammation is thought to play a role in many conditions, including atherosclerosis and heart disease, Alzheimer's disease, and rheumatoid arthritis. In addition, chronic inflammation may play a role in the development of 15 percent of all cancer cases.

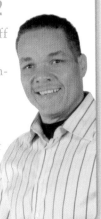

Pete Thomas, Season 2

A lot of parents buy sweet stuff for their families and don't understand that they're poisoning their kids with processed foods. What spells "love" for kids is *time*, not junk food. And with so many overweight kids in our country, tackling that issue starts in the home.

Risk Factors

Smoking is an immunity suppressor. Research has found that long-term exposure to tobacco smoke causes your T cells to function poorly, which may explain why smokers are more likely to develop respiratory infections.

Autoimmune diseases have deeper roots. Because they're more common in women than in men, it is suspected that hormones play a role. For example, women are two to three times more likely

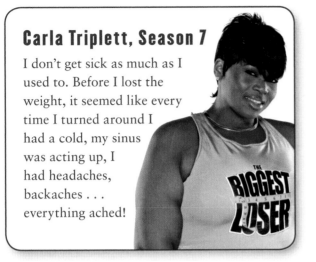

Carla Triplett, Season 7

I don't get sick as much as I used to. Before I lost the weight, it seemed like every time I turned around I had a cold, my sinus was acting up, I had headaches, backaches . . . everything ached!

often causes heat and swelling. The area may become painful, while reaction to the flood of immune cells can include the muscle aches and pains that commonly accompany the onset of an infection.

- **Fever.** Body temperature increases as a protective response to infection and injury. The elevated body temperature (fever) enhances the body's defense mechanisms, although it can cause discomfort. Body temperature is considered elevated when it is higher than 100°F.

The Weight-Loss Connection

Losing weight can help prevent overactive inflammation. In a 2006 study comparing two groups of overweight and obese adults, one group received exercise and diet instruction, and the other didn't participate in any lifestyle changes.

to develop rheumatoid arthritis than men, and more than 90 percent of people with lupus are women. Heredity, too, is a factor.

There's not much you can do change your gender or genetic makeup, but there are things you can do to boost your immune system to keep your defenses strong.

What to Watch For: Monitoring the Defenses

Your body does a good job of letting you know its natural defenses are going to work. The following symptoms often indicate that your immune system is mobilizing for a fight.

- **Inflammation.** As mentioned earlier, the rush of immune cells to a wound or affected area

Heba Salama, Season 6

Ed and I haven't gotten sick at all since we lost the weight, and we both used to get at least the traditional two or three colds a year. Our immune systems are stronger than ever!

The lifestyle-modification group lost weight, improved cholesterol levels, and enjoyed other health benefits. If you're carrying around extra weight, you may be fueling excess inflammation. Cut down your calories and bump up your physical activity.

Ken Coleman of Season 3 used to get sick with colds and general aches and pains about six or seven times a year, if not more. Today, he says he stays healthy year-round. "I've only gotten sick once since I lost weight and got healthy," he remarks. "I feel amazing and have lots of energy to train my clients at the gym. I love showing others that they can do it, too. It's a choice."

Seek Out Vitamin A

Some of your internal body parts interact constantly with the outside world and incoming health threats. Your sinuses, lungs, mouth, and stomach and the rest of your digestive system are lined in a layer of cells called epithelial cells, which are situated close together and covered with a layer of mucus, making it hard for germs to penetrate your system. One of vitamin A's most important jobs is keeping this epithelial barrier strong.

When your diet is deficient in vitamin A, you can develop gaps between epithelial cells, allowing germs to slip through. The recommended daily allowance of vitamin A is 3,000 IU for men and 2,333 IU for women.

Though vitamin A can be found in many animal products (including whole milk and other foods rich in saturated fats), a better place to get vitamin A is from colorful fruits and vegetables. This precursor form is called provitamin A carotenoid, which converts to vitamin A in our bodies. The table below lists several common foods that are abundant in provitamin A.

Food	Serving size	Vitamin A content (IU)
Carrots, cooked, sliced	½ c	13,418
Spinach, cooked	½ c	11,458
Kale, cooked	½ c	9,558
Carrot, raw	7½"	8,666
Cantaloupe, cubed	1 c	5,411
Spinach, raw	1 c	2,813
Papaya, cubed	½ c	766
Mango, sliced	½ c	631
Peach	1 medium	319
Red bell pepper, raw	1 ring, 3" diameter, ¼" thick	313

See to Your C

Is the old wives' tale true—feel a cold coming on, eat an orange? Yes and no. Health experts

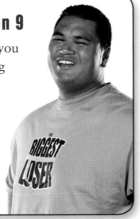
Food	Serving size	Vitamin C content (mg)
Guava	1 medium	165
Red bell pepper	½ c	95
Broccoli, cooked	½ c	60
Orange	1 medium	60
Strawberries	½ c	50
Papaya	½ medium	48
Green bell pepper	½ c	45
Grapefruit, white	½	40
Cantaloupe	½ c	35
Mango	1 medium	30
Cabbage greens, frozen, boiled	½ c	25
Tangerine	1 medium	25
Spinach, raw	1 c	15

have long known that vitamin C plays a crucial role in immunity. The vitamin is present in high concentration in white blood cells. When these cells are low in vitamin C, the deficit is associated with poor immune function. Vitamin C is a powerful antioxidant, preventing free-radical damage to the DNA in your immune system's cells.

Many products marketed as "immunity enhancers" contain megadoses of vitamin C, but the evidence supporting their efficacy is shaky. You're better off getting your vitamin C from your diet. The Recommended Daily Intake (RDI) for vitamin C is 75 milligrams per day, with an upper limit of 2 grams per day. Good sources include the foods in the table on this page.

Boost E and Selenium

Research has found that when your body doesn't get sufficient vitamin E, inflammation tends to be higher, and the immune response to threats is diminished. Adding sources of vitamin E to your diet helps reverse this problem. Vitamin E is also a powerful free-radical-quenching antioxidant, helping to protect your immune system from oxidation. Be sure to get at least 15 milligrams of vitamin E in your diet every day from foods such as the ones in the table on top of page 240.

Food	Serving size	Vitamin E content (mg)
Wheat germ oil	1 Tbsp	20.3
Almonds, dry roasted	2 Tbsp	3.7
Sunflower seed kernels, dry roasted	2 Tbsp	3.0
Hazelnuts, dry roasted	2 Tbsp	2.2
Spinach, cooked	½ c	1.6
Broccoli, cooked	½ c	1.2
Kiwifruit, without skin	1 medium	1.1
Peanuts, dry roasted	2 Tbsp	1.1
Mango, peeled, seeded, and sliced	½ c	0.9
Spinach, raw	1 c	0.6

Selenium is another important player in preventing free radical damage. Not only does sele-nium prevent free radicals from forming, it also stops the chain reaction that results if free radicals begin damaging other molecules. Selenium stimulates the creation of T cells and encourages activity of your immune system's "killer cells." Aim for 55 micrograms of selenium every day. You'll find it in the following foods:

Food	Serving size	Selenium content (mcg)
Brazil nut, dried	1 large	91
Cod, cooked	3 oz	32
Turkey, light meat, roasted	3½ oz	32
Chicken breast, skinless, roasted	3½ oz	20
Egg, whole	1 medium	14
Cottage cheese, fat free	½ c	12
Rice, brown, long grain, cooked	½ c	10
Garlic, chopped	2 Tbsp	3

Think Zinc

A lot of Americans aren't getting enough zinc in their diets. This mineral plays an important role in many immune system activities, and when you don't have enough zinc, you're more susceptible to infection. Evidence from many studies supports the importance of consuming enough zinc. Women

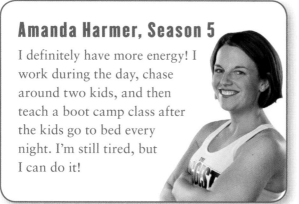

Amanda Harmer, Season 5

I definitely have more energy! I work during the day, chase around two kids, and then teach a boot camp class after the kids go to bed every night. I'm still tired, but I can do it!

should try to get at least 8 milligrams daily, while men should aim for 11 milligrams. You'll find zinc in the following foods:

Food	Serving size	Zinc content (mg)
Oysters, raw	3 medium	16.0
Pork tenderloin, lean only, cooked	3 oz	2.5
Chickpeas, mature seeds, canned	½ c	1.3
Swiss cheese	1 oz	1.1
Chicken breast, skinless, roasted	½	0.9
Milk	1 c	0.9
Mozzarella cheese, low fat, low moisture	1 oz	0.9
Cashews, dry roasted	2 Tbsp	0.8
Kidney beans, California red, cooked	½ c	0.8
Pecans, dry roasted	2 Tbsp	0.7
Mixed nuts with peanuts	2 Tbsp	0.6
Almonds, dry roasted	2 Tbsp	0.5
Flounder or sole, cooked	3 oz	0.5
Walnuts, black, dried	2 Tbsp	0.5

Eat Bacteria—Yes, Bacteria

Probiotics are live bacteria that offer a variety of health benefits, including immune system pro-

tection. Deliberately eating bacteria might seem odd, but many types of yogurt contain bacteria—referred to as "live cultures" on the label—and you probably don't give these invisible ingredients a second thought. Other excellent sources of good bacteria are kefir (a fermented milk drink) and miso, which is found in many Japanese dishes.

Stay Hydrated

Drinking plenty of fluids is important for bringing nutrients and oxygen to your cells and carrying toxins away from them. Make sure you drink at least eight 8-ounce glasses of water each day—and that's in addition to green tea.

Boost Resistance with Exercise

When you're feeling run down, it can be tough to drag yourself to the gym. But believe it or not, exercising—even when you feel like you're "coming down with something"—can help boost your immune response by allowing antibodies and white blood cells to circulate more rapidly in your system. Exercise also increases your body temperature, which may slow down bacterial growth, and reduces levels of stress-related hormones.

Week 6 Menu Plan

MONDAY   1,525 calories

Breakfast

Yogurt smoothie: ¾ cup plain, fat-free Greek-style yogurt; ½ cup unsweetened vanilla almond milk; and ½ cup strawberries

2 ounces smoked salmon or lox

½ whole grain bagel, toasted

Green tea

Snack

2 ounces sliced chicken or turkey breast

¼ cup pumpkin seeds

1 medium apple

Lunch

Biggest Loser BLTE (page 246)

2 cups mixed green salad with 1 medium tomato, sliced, and 1 tablespoon low-fat dressing

1 large wedge cantaloupe

1 cup fat-free milk

Green tea

Snack

⅓ cup hummus

2 medium celery stalks

3 almonds or 6 hazelnuts

Dinner

Broke Bean Stew (page 249) made with kidney beans and kale

½ cup cooked barley

1 cup baby mixed green salad with ¼ avocado, 1 teaspoon extra-virgin olive oil, and 1 teaspoon lemon juice

Green tea

TUESDAY   1,555 calories

Breakfast

Omelet: 1 egg and 3 egg whites filled with ½ cup sautéed onions and mushrooms

2" wedge honeydew melon

1 toasted whole grain English muffin with 2 teaspoons all-fruit spread

1 cup fat-free milk

Green tea

Snack

1 ounce sliced lean turkey breast

3 olives

3 cherry tomatoes

Lunch

1 4-ounce turkey burger on toasted Arnold Sandwich Thin with 2 tomato slices, 2 romaine lettuce leaves, 1 teaspoon Dijon mustard, and 3 slices avocado

2 cups mixed green salad with 1 teaspoon extra-virgin olive oil and 1 teaspoon lemon juice

½ cup fresh berries

Iced green tea

Snack

Shrimp cocktail: 5 large shrimp, boiled or grilled, with ¼ cup cocktail sauce

Dinner

5 ounces sole, baked, with fresh lemon

½ cup cooked barley or brown rice

1 cup steamed broccoli with 1 teaspoon minced garlic and 1 tablespoon chopped walnuts or slivered almonds

1 cup fat-free milk or green tea

WEDNESDAY   1,495 calories

Breakfast

Southern Start (page 71)

2 hard-boiled egg whites

1 cup fresh raspberries

1 cup fat-free milk

Green tea or coffee

Snack

½ cup fat-free cottage cheese topped with 1 tablespoon chopped pumpkin seeds or sunflower seeds and 1 kiwifruit, sliced

Lunch

Out-to-Lunch Tostada Salad (page 251)

1 large apple

Iced tea

Snack

Yogurt smoothie: 1 cup plain, fat-free Greek-style yogurt; ¼ cup mixed berries; ½ banana; and 1 teaspoon ground flaxseed

Dinner

1 cup whole wheat pasta with ½ cup fire-roasted tomatoes, 1 teaspoon garlic, and 1 tablespoon chopped basil

6 ounces halibut, grilled

3 cups baby spinach, wilted

½ cup diced melon and ½ cup fresh berries

Green tea

THURSDAY   1,535 calories

Breakfast

3 slices turkey bacon

½ cup cooked barley with ½ teaspoon ground cinnamon and ¼ cup berries

1 medium wedge cantaloupe

1 cup fat-free milk

Green tea

Snack

1 cup plain, fat-free Greek-style yogurt with
½ teaspoon vanilla extract; ½ banana, sliced;
¼ cup berries; and 2 chopped Brazil nuts
(or 1 tablespoon toasted slivered almonds)

Lunch

2 cups low-fat minestrone soup

1 cup sliced cucumber, ½ cup chopped tomato,
1 tablespoon crumbled low-fat feta cheese,
and 1 tablespoon low-fat dressing

Snack

1½ cups steamed edamame

Dinner

Crab cocktail: 1 cup crabmeat with ½ cup
Avocado Aioli (page 181) or cocktail sauce
served over 3 cups mixed baby greens with
1½ tablespoons low-fat balsamic dressing

1 Wasa cracker

1 cup blueberries with 1 tablespoon chopped
mint

Green tea

FRIDAY   1,555 calories

Breakfast

½ cup cottage cheese topped with
1 tablespoon ground flaxseed

1 cup steel-cut or old-fashioned oatmeal
(cooked in water) with ½ teaspoon ground
cinnamon

1 soft-boiled egg

¼ cup berries

1 cup fat-free milk

Green tea or water

Snack

1 stick low-fat mozzarella cheese

1 apple

3 walnuts

Lunch

Tuna salad sandwich on 2 slices whole grain
bread

4 baby carrots and 1 celery stalk

2 medium tangerines

1 cup fat-free milk

Snack

2 ounces sliced roast turkey or chicken breast

1 tablespoon raw pumpkin seeds

2" wedge honeydew melon

Dinner

5 ounces wild salmon, grilled

½ cup cooked brown rice or whole wheat
couscous

2 cups steamed broccoli raab (or ¾ cup
broccoli and ¾ cup cauliflower, steamed)

¾ cup all-fruit sorbet

SATURDAY   1,565 calories

Breakfast

Cheese omelet: 1 egg and 2 egg whites,
½-ounce slice reduced-fat provolone cheese,
¼ teaspoon dry or 1 teaspoon fresh thyme,
and 2 slices Canadian bacon, diced

2" wedge cantaloupe

1 cup fat-free milk

Green tea or coffee

Snack

1 large apple, sliced, with 1 tablespoon almond
butter or peanut butter

Lunch

1 serving **Fire-Roasted Tomato Soup** (page 252)

½ grilled cheese sandwich: 1 sliced reduced-fat
Cheddar cheese and 1 teaspoon Dijon
mustard on 1 slice whole grain bread

1 cup red grapes

Iced tea

Snack

¼ cup hummus

1 celery stalk

Dinner

Cheesy Stuffed Chicken Breast (page 255)

1 cup steamed brussels sprouts

½ small roasted sweet potato

Green tea or coffee

SUNDAY   1,515 calories

Breakfast

1 cup Kashi GoLean cereal

¾ cup fat-free milk

½ banana, sliced, and ¼ cup fresh berries

4 slices turkey bacon

Green tea or coffee

Snack

2-ounce slice lean turkey or chicken breast

¼ cup fresh cherries or berries

3 almonds

Lunch

My German Lover (page 256)

2 cups mixed green salad with 1 tablespoon
low-fat Caesar dressing

½ cup cubed melon

1 cup fat-free milk

Snack

½ cup fat-free cottage cheese or ricotta topped
with 1 teaspoon flaxseed and ¼ cup berries

Dinner

6 ounces halibut, grilled

1 red bell pepper, roasted

3 cups baby spinach, wilted, with 1 teaspoon
balsamic vinegar, 1 teaspoon grated
Parmesan cheese, and ground black pepper

½ cup fat-free frozen yogurt with ¼ cup
blueberries and 1 tablespoon toasted pecans

BIGGEST LOSER BLTE

Season 7's Carla Triplett created this high-protein version of her favorite sandwich, a twist on the classic BLT. When she's really watching her carbs, she serves it open-face style, on one piece of bread.

2 slices Ezekiel whole wheat bread

3 slices Trader Joe's turkey bacon

2 tablespoons spicy mustard

1 wedge Laughing Cow Light French Onion cheese

½ cup egg whites or 1 whole egg

2 tomato slices

1 leaf green leaf lettuce

Toast the bread. Cook the turkey bacon, then cut the strips in half.

Mix the mustard with the cheese and spread on the toast.

In a nonstick skillet coated with cooking oil spray, cook the egg as desired. Place the lettuce, bacon, egg, and tomatoes on the cheese-covered toast. Cut in half and serve immediately.

Makes 1 sandwich

Per serving: 340 calories, 34 g protein, 35 g carbohydrates (2 g sugars), 5 g fat (1 g saturated), 40 mg cholesterol, 8 g fiber, 420 mg sodium

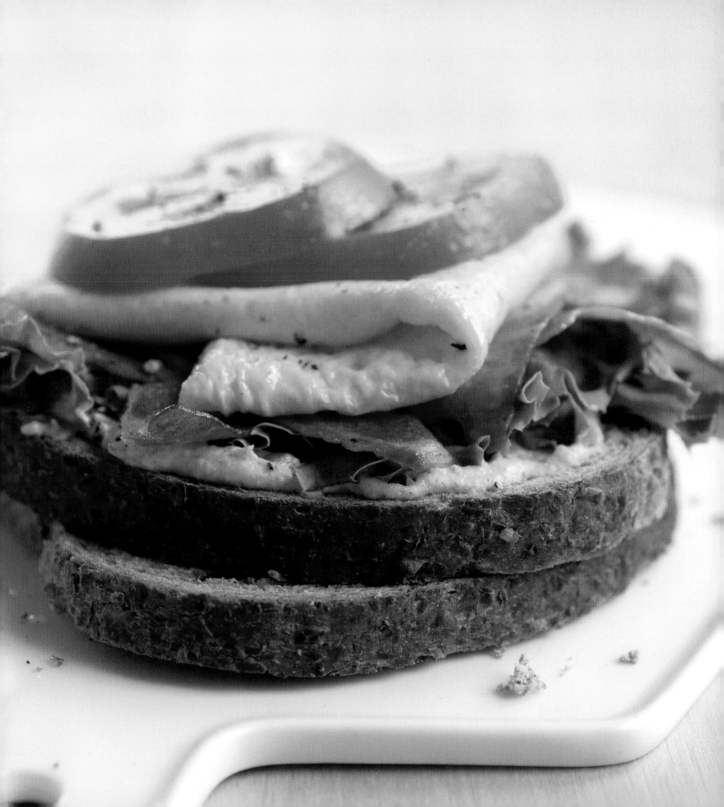

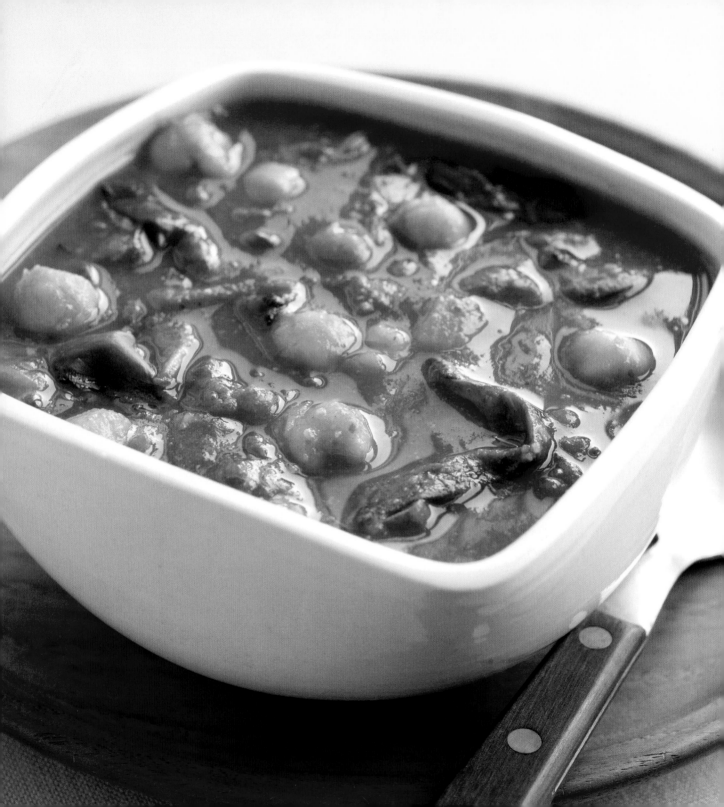

BROKE BEAN STEW

Season 4's Nicole Michalik says, "I love, love, love this recipe! It's high in protein but totally vegetarian! It's so easy to make and freezes very well. I make it at least once a month." Beans are a great, inexpensive source of protein and fiber. This hearty stew makes a satisfying meal, especially in the colder months.

1 tablespoon olive oil

1 large yellow or white onion, chopped

1 tablespoon chopped garlic

1 (28-ounce) can diced fire-roasted tomatoes

1 teaspoon ground cumin

1 teaspoon chili powder

1 teaspoon red chile flakes (optional)

3 (15½-ounce) cans chickpeas, kidney beans, black beans, or white beans, rinsed and drained, or 4½ cups cooked beans

4 cups fat-free, low-sodium chicken or vegetable broth

¼ cup chopped cilantro

3 cups fresh baby spinach leaves or 3 cups chopped kale or Swiss chard

In a 4-quart saucepan, heat the oil over medium-high heat. Add the onion and cook for about 5 minutes, until softened but not browned. Add the garlic and cook for 1 minute longer. Do not brown the garlic.

Add the tomatoes, cumin, chili powder, and chile flakes, if desired. Simmer for about 5 minutes. Add 3 cups (2 cans) of the beans and 3½ cups of the broth and bring to a boil. Reduce to a simmer.

Meanwhile, place the remaining 1½ cups of beans and ½ cup of broth in a food processor or blender. Add the cilantro and puree or blend until smooth.

Add the puree to the stew. Add the greens and heat just until wilted. Stir well and serve hot.

Makes 10 (1-cup) servings

Per serving: 160 calories, 8 g protein, 26 g carbohydrates (7 g sugars), 3 g fat (0 g saturated), 0 mg cholesterol, 7 g fiber, 330 mg sodium

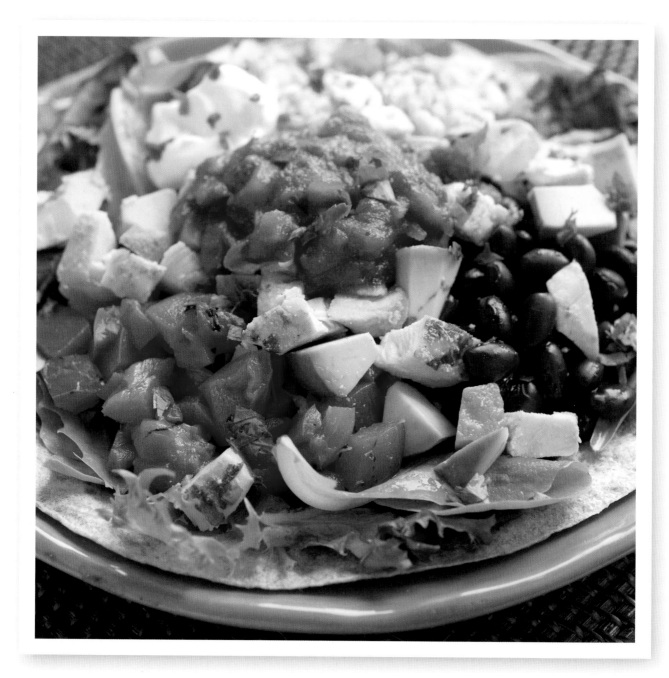

OUT-TO-LUNCH TOSTADA SALAD

My trips to The Biggest Loser *Ranch allowed me to spend downtime with the contestants, during which I could teach them about nutrition and cooking, take them on grocery store tours, and show them how to make healthy choices while dining out. This salad is a rendition of one of the contestants' favorites from a Mexican restaurant near the Ranch. It is loaded with fiber and protein and is very filling.*

1 whole wheat tortilla

2 cups baby lettuce mix

¼ cup cooked brown rice

¼ cup cooked black beans

½ cup fire-roasted sliced bell peppers, diced

4 ounces grilled chicken breast, diced

¼ avocado, diced

½ cup low-sodium salsa

1 tablespoon plain, fat-free Greek-style yogurt

2 tablespoons chopped cilantro

Toast the tortilla in a toaster oven until crisp. Place the lettuce mix on the tortilla. Then, in clockwise fashion, top the lettuce with the rice, beans, and bell peppers. Sprinkle the chicken and avocado on top. Place a spoonful of salsa in the center and top with a dollop of yogurt. Garnish with the cilantro.

Makes 1 serving

Per serving: 400 calories, 39 g protein, 44 g carbohydrates (2 g sugars), 11 g fat (9 g saturated), 65 mg cholesterol, 18 g fiber, 310 mg sodium

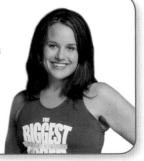

Nicole Michalik, Season 4

Try making a superfood salad with acai/gogi berries, wheat berries, spinach, kale, tomatoes, onions, olive oil, and balsamic vinegar. So amazing!

FIRE-ROASTED TOMATO SOUP

America's all-time favorite comfort soup is jazzed up with the addition of flavorful fire-roasted tomatoes and aromatic, spicy ginger. Tomatoes—especially when cooked—are full of cancer-fighting lycopene, and ginger is thought to aid in digestion.

1 teaspoon olive oil

2 tablespoons minced shallot or onion

4 quarter-size slices peeled fresh ginger

1 tablespoon chopped garlic

1½ cups (14½-ounce can) diced fire-roasted tomatoes

1 cup fat-free chicken or vegetable broth

½ cup 1% or fat-free milk

Salt and ground black pepper to taste

1 tablespoon chopped fresh chives or scallion

In a 2-quart saucepan, heat the oil over medium heat. Add the shallot or onion and ginger and cook until softened, about 1 minute.

Add the garlic and tomatoes to the saucepan. Simmer for about 4 minutes, until the mixture begins to thicken. Add the broth and milk and just bring to a boil.

Carefully transfer the soup to a food processor or blender. Process or blend until smooth. Return to the saucepan and serve immediately. Add salt and pepper to taste and garnish with the chives or scallion.

Makes 4 (¾-cup) servings, or 3 cups

Per serving: 60 calories, 2 g protein, 8 g carbohydrates (5 g sugars), 2 g fat (0 g saturated), 0 mg cholesterol, 2 g fiber, 360 mg sodium

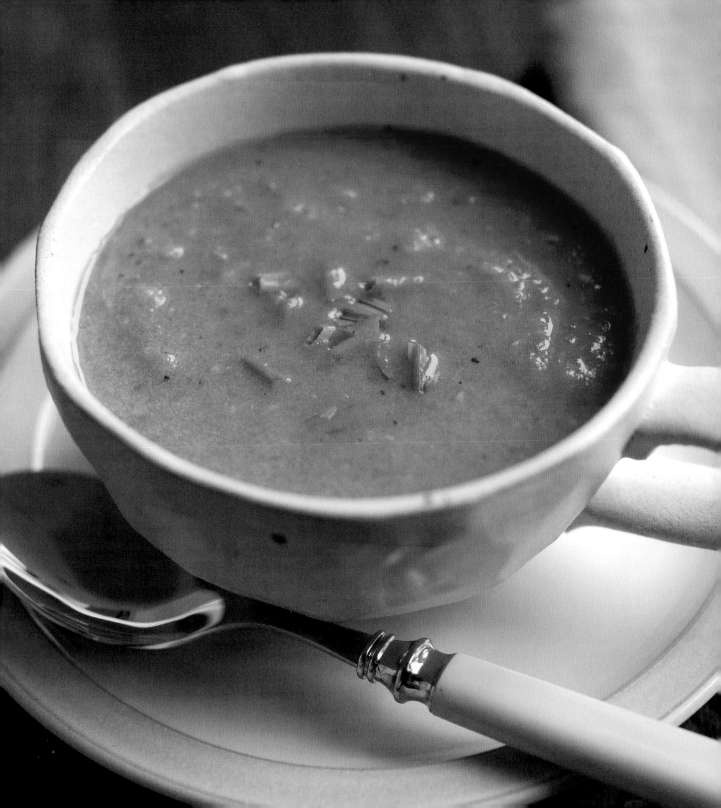

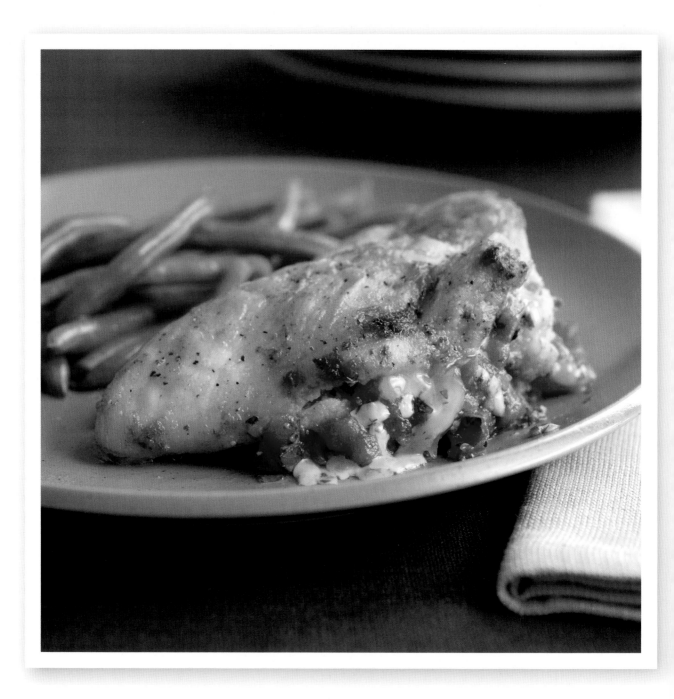

CHEESY STUFFED CHICKEN BREAST

This scrumptious main course is surprisingly easy to prepare, though it will look as if you've spent hours cooking. That makes it perfect for company! Feel free to experiment with different low-fat cheeses and fresh herbs.

¼ cup (1 ounce) shredded low-fat Monterey Jack cheese

½ cup diced fire-roasted tomatoes

½ teaspoon red chile flakes (optional)

2 tablespoons chopped cilantro + extra for garnish

½ teaspoon salt

4 (4-ounce) boneless, skinless chicken breasts

3 tablespoons white whole wheat flour

¼ teaspoon ground black pepper

2 teaspoons olive oil

In a small bowl, combine the cheese, tomatoes, chile flakes (if desired), 2 tablespoons cilantro, and ¼ teaspoon of the salt.

Place 1 chicken breast on a cutting board and hold it flat with your hand. Using a slender, sharp knife, carefully cut a horizontal pocket in the side of the breast, making the pocket as large as you can without cutting through the other side. Repeat for the remaining chicken breasts. Spoon ¼ of the cheese-tomato mixture into each pocket and close the pocket with a toothpick.

In a shallow dish, combine the flour, black pepper, and remaining ¼ teaspoon salt. Dredge the stuffed chicken into the flour mixture, coating on all sides.

In a large nonstick skillet, heat the oil over medium-high heat. Add the chicken and cook just until tender, about 4 minutes per side. Remove the toothpicks and garnish with cilantro. Serve immediately.

Makes 4 servings

Per serving: 200 calories, 27 g protein, 7 g carbohydrates (1 g sugars), 7 g fat (2 g saturated), 70 mg cholesterol, 1 g fiber, 375 mg sodium

MY GERMAN LOVER

Season 9's Andrea Hough loves to make this sandwich in the morning and keep it in the fridge for later, when she warms it up on The Biggest Loser *panini press for a quick postworkout snack. If you prefer, you can substitute sliced lean turkey or chicken for the beef.*

1 tablespoon German mustard (see note)

2 slices Ezekiel whole grain bread

½ wedge Laughing Cow Light Garlic and Herb cheese

2½ ounces extra-lean, low-sodium sliced roast beef

2 slices medium red onion

Ground black pepper and salt substitute to taste

Preheat a panini press to medium.

Spread the mustard on 1 slice of bread and place the cheese on the other slice. Arrange the roast beef and onion between the slices of bread, seasoning as desired with pepper and salt substitute.

Place the assembled sandwich on the press and cook for about 3 minutes, or until the bread is toasted and the sandwich hot. Cut in half and serve immediately.

Note: German mustards come in several styles: mild, hot, sweet, and spicy. Although Andrea favors a hot German mustard, you can use your own favorite.

Makes 1 sandwich

Per serving: 270 calories, 23 g protein, 36 g carbohydrates (1 g sugars), 4 g fat (< 1 g saturated), 10 mg cholesterol, 6 g fiber, 600 mg sodium

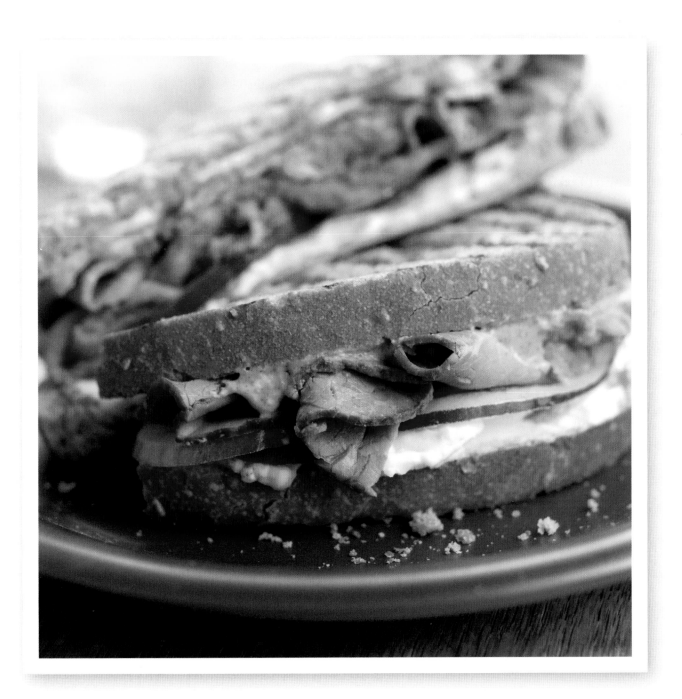

Week 6 Exercises

Exercise improves your mood, helps you handle stress, and promotes better sleep. It provides an immunity boost—it helps antibodies and white blood cells circulate more rapidly in your body and reduces the number of stress-related hormones present in your system.

Keep in mind, though, that if you are really sick or recovering from a serious illness, working out might do more harm than good. Overly intense exercise can raise your blood pressure and release certain hormones that can suppress your immune system. If you are feeling healthy, pick up the pace and intensity level to boost your immune system. But if you're a bit under the weather, take it down a notch.

Pilates is a comprehensive system of core-based exercises designed by Joseph Pilates in 1912. The guiding principles include centering, alignment, control, concentration/focus, precision, breathing, and flow/integration. Not only will Pilates help you develop a strong core, it will also dynamically stretch and balance the muscles of your legs and upper body.

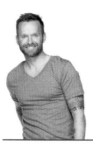

Biggest Loser Trainer Tip: Bob Harper

A bike is a great thing to own to stay healthy. Instead of driving everywhere, try biking. When you start, warm up for 5 minutes. Once you get your heart rate up, keep it there for at least 20 minutes. When you've finished, go at a slow, steady pace for another 5 minutes. It's effective and something you'll never forget—just like riding a bike!

Focus: Pilates
Workout Guidelines

- For this program, all you need is a mat or carpeted surface. This great core workout focuses on flexion, extension, rotation, and stabilization.
- Warm up the muscles around your spine with a simple Cat Cow motion from yoga. Begin on all fours with your shoulders over your hands and your hips over your knees. Inhale and arch your back, tilting your head and tailbone up to the ceiling. Exhale and round your back. Repeat for about 30 seconds.
- Concentrate on breathing throughout the exercises. Don't hold your breath!
- Focus on correct alignment, technique, and form rather than repetitions. It's better to do fewer repetitions with precision and better form.
- Perform the recommended repetitions for one set of each exercise for one full circuit of five exercises. As you get stronger, build up to three circuits.
- Begin with the most basic variation. As you get stronger, work up to the intermediate and advanced progressions.
- Use the workout on its own for a quick core workout on busy days. For greater results, add one to three circuits of these exercises to any and all of the previous weeks workouts to add time, variation, and intensity. As an example of a well-rounded weekly program, try the cardio workout plus Pilates session 4 days a week, the strength/resistance and/or circuit workout plus Pilates session 2 days a week, and the restorative yoga session once a week.
- If you have any spinal injuries, suffer from sciatica or recently had abdominal surgery (including C-section), please consult a physician before beginning this program.

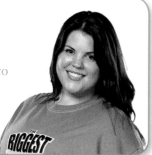

Stephanie Anderson, Season 9

Keep workouts fun and learn to use as many of the machines at the gym as possible. When I first came to the Ranch, I was afraid of the StairMaster. But no longer. And now that I learned Spinning, it's what I'm going to incorporate into my routine at home.

SINGLE-LEG STRETCH

Lie on your back on a mat or carpeted surface. Bend your knees and lift your legs and feet, so your shins are parallel to the floor. Slowly curl your torso to lift your head and shoulders off the floor, keeping your spine flexed and placing your hands on your shins. Extend your left leg to the point of control while placing your left hand on your right leg below the knee and your right hand on your shin. Hold for 2 seconds, then, maintaining a stable pelvis, switch legs and hands and hold again. That's 1 repetition. Do 8 to 10 repetitions.

Tips

- Drop your shoulders down and back.
- Avoid any rocking or movement of your hips and torso.

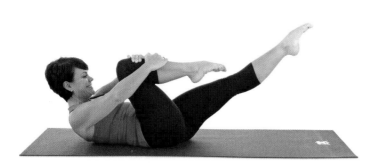

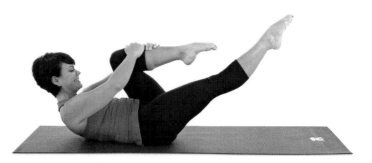

Intermediate Progression

Lower your leg closer to the floor.

Advanced Progression

Place your hands behind your head.

CRISSCROSS

Lie on your back on a mat or carpeted surface. Bend your knees and lift your legs and feet, so your shins are parallel to the floor. Slowly curl your torso to lift your head and shoulders off the floor, keeping your spine flexed and your hands behind your head. Extend your left leg to the point of control and cross your left shoulder toward your right knee. Hold for 2 seconds, then, maintaining a stable pelvis, switch legs and shoulders and hold again. That's 1 repetition. Do 8 to 10 repetitions.

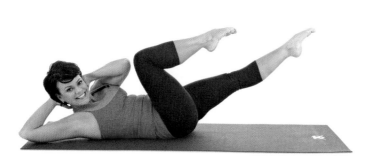

Tips

- Drop your shoulders down and back.
- Avoid any rocking or movement of your hips and torso.
- Keep your chest open and draw the bottom of your rib cage to the opposite hip.

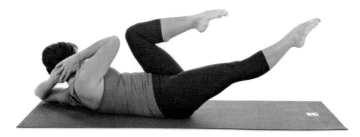

Intermediate Progression
Lower your leg closer to the floor.

Advanced Progression
Straighten both legs.

SWIMMING

Lie on your belly on a mat or carpeted surface with your legs and arms extended so your body's in one straight line. Engage your abdominals and lift your arms and legs so that you extend your spine and hips. Begin a "swimming" flutter motion by lifting your right leg and left arm higher, then lowering them as you lift your left leg and right arm higher. Repeat for five full breaths (about 30 seconds).

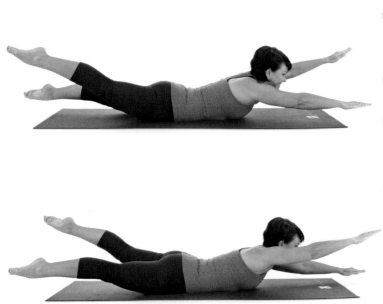

Tips

- To avoid compressing your lower back, imagine lengthening out as opposed to lifting up.
- Draw in your abdominals during the entire exercise.
- Drop your shoulders down and back and keep your head in line with your spine.
- Avoid any rocking or movement of your hips and torso.

Intermediate Progression

Make the movements larger.

Advanced Progression

Alternate internally and externally rotating at the shoulders (moving thumbs up or thumbs down).

FRONT AND BACK

Lie on your left side on a mat or carpeted surface. Form one line from the crown of your head to your hips and extend your legs slightly forward. Rest your head on your left arm and place your right hand on the floor in front of you for support. Flex your foot and hip to bring your right leg forward. Pulse the leg upward two times, then point your foot and extend the same leg behind you. Do 6 to 8 repetitions, then roll over and perform the exercise with your left leg.

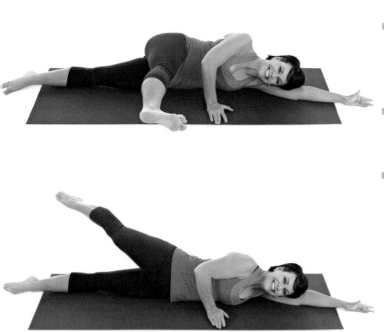

Tips

- Reach out through your heel when your leg is forward and reach through your toes when your leg is extended back.
- Keep your hips stacked during the entire range of motion; avoid any rocking or tilting of your pelvis.
- Don't allow your back to round or arch. The only movement should be in the raised leg and hip.

Intermediate Progression

Lift up onto the elbow of the arm that's on the floor, into a slight side bend.

Advanced Progression

Place your hands behind your head.

LEG PULLUP

Begin in a reverse plank position: Facing the ceiling, support your weight on your hands and feet only, with your hips lifted, your hands under your shoulders, and your feet pointed. Tuck your chin, engage your core, and lift your right leg up toward the ceiling, keeping your hips lifted and shoulders pulled down and away from your ears. Hold for 2 seconds, then lower your leg. Repeat with your left leg. Continue alternating for 6 to 8 reps with each leg.

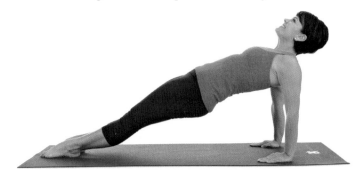

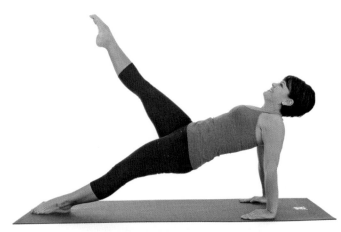

Tips

- As you lift your leg, avoid arching or rounding your back; keep your hips level.
- Your fingers should be pointing toward your hips.
- Keep your ribs "soft" and press your hands into the floor so that your shoulders stay down and away from your ears.
- Imagine your hips being suspended from the ceiling.
- To make the move a little easier, lift your leg only a few inches off the floor.

Intermediate Progression
Look up at the ceiling and keep your head in line with your spine.

Advanced Progression
Increase the range of motion and/or open your leg out to the side.

Rebecca Meyer, Season 8

When you're upset about something, instead of taking a nap or hitting the refrigerator, hit a boxing bag instead! Go take it out in an hour at the gym. You will feel so much better! All those endorphins really do help.

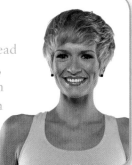

Cathy Skell, Season 7

Since I have lost weight, my asthma has really improved. Many people around me have gotten colds, but I manage to stay healthy. And I just turned 50! I have never felt better and happier in my life. My asthma barely flares up anymore, which is amazing.

Abby Rike, Season 8

I love hiking. Being in the fresh air and beautiful scenery and climbing a mountain is good for your soul. When you get to your destination, you have such a sense of accomplishment.

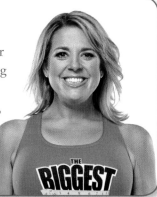

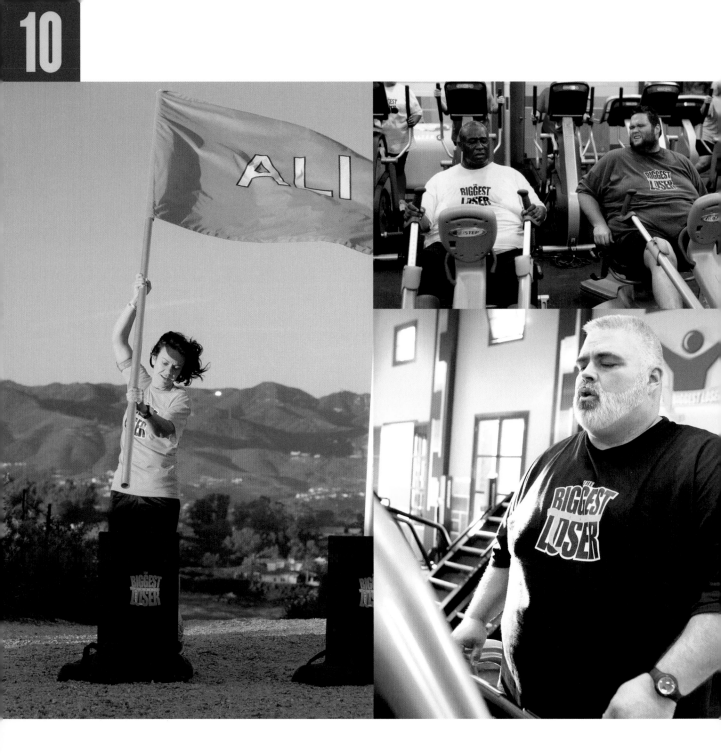

10

A Healthier You for Life

Now that you have all the tools to live your healthiest, happiest life, it's just a matter of day-to-day vigilance. Weight loss can be dramatic and exciting, especially if you have a lot to lose. It can even be lifesaving, as we've seen from many of the stories in this book. But for many people, it will be more subtle—you may suddenly realize you're not as tired as usual at 5:00 in the evening. You might find yourself able to participate in new activities with friends and family. Maybe your digestion improves, you get sick less often, or you get fewer headaches. These are not showstopping changes, but they add up to a vastly improved quality of life.

Over time, you'll know exactly what works for you and why. The plan in this book is a good place to start. Eventually, though, you should personalize it to fit your life. You might want to follow the recommended calorie count for each day but swap some foods for others. Or you may experiment with the recipes to create a new favorite. Or

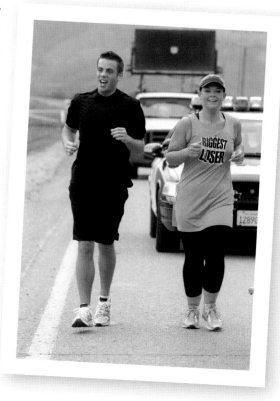

maybe you prefer to mix the body-weight training in week 1 with the cardio and strength-training exercises in week 4. Pay attention to what feels right for you. And of course, you'll always get truthful feedback from occasional check-ins with the scale or your clothes. If the number is inching up or your jeans are feeling a bit too tight, something's out of whack. Figure out why before you get too far off track.

There are some things you'll always have to do, no matter how healthy you get or how great you feel. When Season 5 winner Ali Vincent visited the Season 9 contestants at the Ranch, she was deluged with questions about "how she did it" and how she kept it going once she returned home.

"You have to plan," she told Vicky and Cherita Andrews, who ended up going home after week 1. "Everything they taught you and that you've heard and read, absorb that. Eat every 3 to 4 hours. Log your food and exercise. It's a mathematical equation.

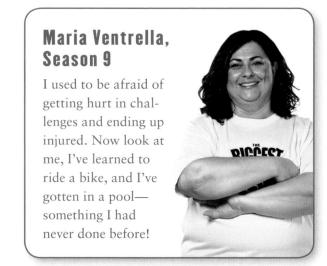

Maria Ventrella, Season 9

I used to be afraid of getting hurt in challenges and ending up injured. Now look at me, I've learned to ride a bike, and I've gotten in a pool—something I had never done before!

It's calories in, calories out. Get your goal on paper. Write down how much weight you want to lose and calculate how long it's going to take to lose it. Ask for support from friends and family. Tell them how they can support you—so it doesn't feel like you're being policed, so you don't start hiding. Figure out how you got here. I made a choice to stay conscious and present; to live and breathe in the moment; to write down my food, my issues, my exercise; to think."

The most important thing Ali says she's learned in the 2 years she's been living a healthy life is the ability to forgive herself. "Now, if I make a bad

Biggest Loser Trainer Tip: Jillian Michaels

True or false: Does snacking inhibit weight loss?
The answer is false. Nutritionists recommend that people plan snacks into their day. Smart snacking may curb hunger and prevent overeating at meals. The key is knowing how many calories are in your snacks and choosing snacks with nutrients, such as fruits, whole grains and nuts and protein.

choice, I quickly move on. I don't waste time beating myself up, not anymore," she says.

But she still holds herself accountable every day. "If I don't feel it when I work out, I know I need to step it up a notch. I think it's just a matter of being conscious. I don't *have* to do anything. I *choose* to do it."

A Delicate Balance

It's a fine balance, tweaking your plan but not kidding yourself about the effort you're making over time. "There's an element of honesty in losing weight," says Sean Algaier of Season 8. "Every day, you do your best. If you go to bed and you're unhappy with yourself, that's a big red flag."

Before *The Biggest Loser*, Sean said he had lost consciousness about himself and his role as a father and a husband. "Now I'm aware. I've gained accountability. You can only live with so much guilt, and I've lost the guilt. I went on a personal journey of anguish and grief—and I came out on the other side."

Keep Talking

Don't forget your support system! As Pete Thomas of Season 2 suggests, make your spouse your partner. He teaches this in his weight-loss classes back in Michigan. "Keep a handwritten contract between the two of you and spell out how you need him or her to work with you. If your spouse needs to eat food you don't want around the house, ask them to eat it away from you, when they are out of the house. Or they can keep their food in a particular cabinet in the kitchen, a cabinet that you, in turn, promise to avoid."

Jerry and Estella Hayes of Season 7 find that talking to others, including groups, is a way to keep their own batteries recharged. "My sister has started losing weight, my daughter has lost more than 80 pounds, and now my 88-year-old mom asks questions during family dinners, such as 'What do you eat?' and 'How do you fix your

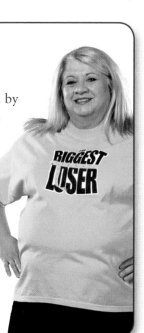

Sherry Johnston, Season 9

I used to be intimidated by all the equipment in the gym. But get a trainer to show you how to use just a couple of machines. Most gyms have someone on the floor who knows how things work. That's what they're there for, to help you. Ask for help!

The Real Cost of Obesity

When financial guru Suze Orman visited the Season 8 contestants at the Ranch, she tested their knowledge of the financial implications their unhealthy lifestyles could create. Test yourself with the questions below and see if you know how much an unhealthy lifestyle could cost you down the road.

1. Research shows that obese employees earn less money than their fellow workers. On average, how much less do obese employees make in 1 year?

   A. $700

   B. $7,000

   C. $17,000

2. How much can a family of four save in a year by swapping one meal out for one at home every day?

   A. $876

   B. $8,760

   C. $18,760

3. How much do Americans spend on obesity-related health issues each year?

   A. $14.7 million

   B. $1.47 billion

   C. $147 billion

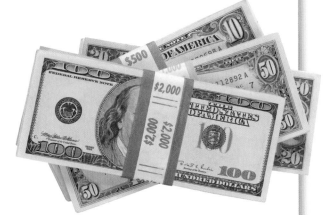

food?' " says Estella. "We have gained knowledge from this life-changing experience, and we continue to pass it on."

Appreciate Your Gains

Don't ever lose sight of what you gain each day: more energy, a brighter outlook, and, over time, maybe something even bigger—for Season 7's Laura Denoux, a boyfriend! "Before *The Biggest Loser,* I would stay at home all the time because I was ashamed of how I looked," she says. "I was one of those 'pretty fat girls' who had not been asked for her phone number or been out on a date since gaining weight.

"I never told anyone this," she adds, "but before going on the show, I started to fall in love with one of my male friends, Nick. Being overweight held me back from dating, which is devastating to a young 25-year-old woman. When I got eliminated from the show in February 2009, I came home and told Nick how I felt. He felt the same way. . . . Now we are in love!"

The love-struck Laura continues, "If I hadn't lost this weight, I would have never had the opportunity to express my feelings to him. I could not be happier. I have lost the weight, and I feel great about myself not only physically but mentally. I figured out who I am. I have now found a new body, new love, a new *me!*"

Make Time for Yourself

One thing you should never skimp on in this process—and for the rest of your life—is you. It's crucial that you set aside adequate time for yourself. Don't let distractions consistently drive you away from what you need most to be healthy and active. Season 5's Amanda Harmer, who is a mother of two young children, says, "I used to make excuse after excuse. But once you make up your mind to lose weight, nothing will get in your way. Always make the time to take care of yourself, whether good things or bad are going on. I make sure I have time in my day to prepare great food and exercise. It's just that important to me."

Sure, making time in a packed schedule can be

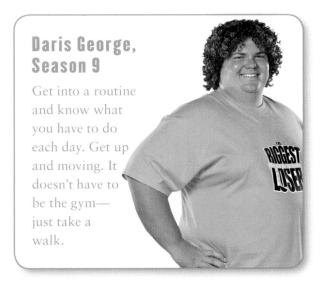

Daris George, Season 9

Get into a routine and know what you have to do each day. Get up and moving. It doesn't have to be the gym— just take a walk.

hard. But so what? It's simply something you have to do. "We all have to work hard to lose the weight," says Alexandra White of Season 8. "Whether you're on the Ranch or not—you really have to dig deep. That's one thing I've learned. I feel extremely firm and committed just because I've been doing this for the past 7 months. It really has become a lifestyle; it's nothing temporary. Exercise and eating healthy are now part of my life."

Look Forward to Your Future

The one thing all *Biggest Loser* contestants gain from getting healthy is a future. Bill Germanakos, the grand prize winner of Season 4, says, "Two and a half years ago, if you had asked me about my future, it would not have included being a motivational speaker. Now if you ask me about my future, I think it's bright. I'm looking forward to walking my two daughters down the aisle. I'm looking for-ward to meeting, greeting, and spoiling some grandkids. I never could have said that when I weighed 334 pounds."

Bernie Salazar of Season 5 says he wants to help make sure kids get a healthy future, too. "Losing weight gave me my life back. In fact, it gave me a *better* life back, better than I really expected. I want to make sure I'm paying it back. Childhood obesity rates in this country are ridiculous. We're facing an epidemic that can be reversed, and I plan on being on the forefront of that."

Bernie has written an interactive children's book called *Monstercise*, which is all about get-ting kids up and out of their chairs and dancing along with an imaginary monster. A teacher by trade, Bernie is visiting schools across the coun-try, reading his book aloud, and getting kids to giggle and play a bit.

Season 7's Helen Phillips and Season 5 winner Ali Vincent are also involved in local campaigns to help kids reach for a brighter, healthier future.

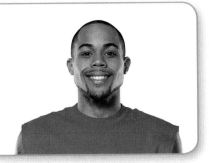

Antoine Dove, Season 8

At work, I am much more productive because I'm not tired all the time. In the gym, I have a lot more energy to push myself to new limits and do exercises that I would have never dreamed of doing before *The Biggest Loser*. All around, I feel like I am the human version of the Energizer Bunny!

Helen works with local schools to teach kids how to make good food choices, and Ali is working with local children's hospitals on obesity awareness programs.

Don't forget, a spirit of gratitude will surround you when you get healthy. Pete Thomas joined a group of past *Biggest Loser* contestants for a half-marathon in San Francisco in July 2009. Even years after his season was complete, Thomas says, "I'm really thankful I can do things I never thought I'd be able to do. I never thought I'd be able to run 13.1 miles. I never thought I'd be able to run *3* miles." One of his co-runners, Carla Triplett of Season 7, adds, "I feel like a million bucks right now, like I'm sitting on top of the world."

So stick to your journey, get and stay healthy, and reach for your goals. A healthier you starts with the choices you make today.

Michael Ventrella, Season 9

Each day, you are going to feel better than the one before. You will move better, you will not be as tired, you will enjoy a little more of each day. Developing a healthy mind and body will become addictive, will help you develop a more positive outlook on life. Strive to do and be better than who you were the day before. It's just plain and simple.

References

Chiasson, M. D. "Evidence-Based Nutrition Principles and Recommendations for the Treatment and Prevention of Diabetes and Related Complications," *Diabetes Care* 25, no. 1 (January 2002): 202–212; Martin, J., "Chromium Picolinate Supplementation Attenuates Body Weight Gain and Increases Insulin Sensitivity in Subjects with Type 2 Diabetes," *Diabetes Care* 29, no. 8 (August 2006): 1826–32.

Field, Catherine J., Ian R. Johnson, and Patricia D. Schley. "Nutrients and Their Role in Host Resistance to Infection.," *Journal of Leukoc Biology* 71, no. 1 (January 2002): 16–32.

Fox, Caroline S., MD, MPH, et al. "Trends in the Incidence of Type 2 Diabetes Mellitus from the 1970s to the 1990s," Framingham Heart Study, *Circulation* 113 (2006): 2914–2918, http://www.circ.ahajournals.org/cgi/content/abstract/113/25/2914.

Heilbronn, L. K., and E. Ravussin. "Calorie Restriction and Aging: Review of the Literature and Implications for Studies in Humans," *American Journal of Clinical Nutrition* 78 (2003): 361–69.

Hu, Frank B., MD, et al. "Diet, Lifestyle, and the Risk of Type 2 Diabetes Mellitus in Women," *New England Journal of Medicine* 13, vol. 11 (September 2001): 790–97.

Jae, S. Y., et al. "Effects of Lifestyle Modifications on C-Reactive Protein: Contribution of Weight Loss and Improved Aerobic Capacity," *Metabolism* 55, vol. 6 (June 2006): 825–31.

Sakara, Devan, and Paul B. Fisher. "Molecular Mechanisms of Aging-Associated Inflammation," *Cancer Letters* 236, vol. 1 (2006 May): 13–23; Marx J. "Inflammation and Cancer: The Link Grows Stronger," *Science* 306, no. 5698 (November 5, 2004): 966–68.

Simopoulos, A. P., "Omega-3 Fatty Acids in Inflammation and Autoimmune Diseases," *Journal of the American College of Nutrition* 21, no. 6 (2002): 495–505.

Spence, J. David. Nutrition and Stroke Prevention, http://www.americanheart.org/presenter.jhtml?identifier=535.

Resources

The following Web sites provide more detailed information about the chronic diseases mentioned in this book, and what you can do to prevent them.

Diabetes

www.diabetes.org

www.nlm.nih.gov

diabetes.niddk.nih.gov

www.cdc.gov/diabetes/projects/cda2.htm

Heart Disease and High Blood Pressure

www.americanheart.org

www.cdc.gov/heartdisease

www.mayoclinic.com/health

www.hsph.harvard.edu/nutritionsource/what-should-you-eat/fats-and-cholesterol

Cancer

www.cancer.org

www.cancer.gov

http://www.mayoclinic.com/health/cancer/DS01076

www.nlm.nih.gov/medlineplus/ency/article/002439.htm

Cognitive Health

www.alz.org

www.nia.nih.gov/Alzheimers/Publications

www.nlm.nih.gov/medlineplus/depression.html

http://www.mayoclinic.com/health/dementia/DS01131

Immunity

www.cdc.gov/h1n1flu/in_the_news.htm

www.hsph.harvard.edu/nutritionsource/what-should-you-eat

http://dietary-supplements.info.nih.gov

Contributors

CHERYL FORBERG, RD, is the nutritionist for NBC's *The Biggest Loser,* for which she codeveloped the eating plan.

A James Beard Award–winning chef, Cheryl received her culinary education at the California Culinary Academy (CCA) in San Francisco. After graduating from CCA, she embarked on a European apprenticeship at top French restaurants. Upon returning to the United States, Cheryl was part of the opening team for Postrio, Wolfgang Puck's first venture in northern California.

Cheryl earned her Nutrition and Clinical Dietetics degree and RD certification from the University of California at Berkeley. Her writing and recipes have appeared in such publications as *Health,* the *Washington Post,* and *Prevention,* for which she is on the advisory board. She is a *New York Times* best-selling author who has written or contributed to 13 books. Cheryl is a speaker, teacher, and spokesperson and writes a weekly blog of cooking and nutrition tips at cherylforberg.com. She lives in Napa, California.

MELISSA ROBERSON is the editor of BiggestLoserClub.com, the Web site that offers customized food and fitness plans and inspiration to Biggest Losers everywhere. She is a coauthor of the *New York Times* bestsellers *The Biggest Loser Family Cookbook, The Biggest Loser 30-Day Jump Start,* and *The Biggest Loser Simple Swaps.* She lives in Hoboken, New Jersey.

LISA WHEELER is a consultant for *The Biggest Loser,* an international dance/fitness professional, and the national creative manager for Equinox. She is the choreographer for Lionsgate Films and Cal Pozo's Fit Vid Productions, where her clients include *The Biggest Loser, Dancing with the Stars,* Jillian Michaels, and Denise Austin. Lisa has starred in more than 20 fitness videos, leads the Westin Workout segments on SPG TV, and has hosted fitness programs for Fit TV, the NFL Channel, *CNN Headline News, The View,* and QVC. Lisa is also a contributing editor to *Shape* magazine. She lives in New York City.

Acknowledgments

Cheryl Forberg

To my coauthor and very close friend, Melissa Roberson, it is such a joy to work with you. I look forward to many more projects (and adventures!) together. And to Lisa Wheeler—thanks for all of your great work on these books.

To everyone at NBC and Reveille—executives, producers, and crew of *The Biggest Loser,* especially Mark Koops and Chad Bennett—thank you for all the opportunities! I also want to thank Kat Elmore and Julie Ann Harris for making my visits and communiqués to the Ranch so seamless. Thank you to trainers Bob Harper and Jillian Michaels, who dedicate themselves tirelessly to the contestants and to the show.

To my peers on *The Biggest Loser* Medical Expert Team, Dr. Rob Huizenga, Dr. Michael Dansinger, Dr. Sean Hogan, and Sandy Krum: Thanks so much for all your guidance and support.

Thanks to Catherine Thorpe for your creativity, brilliant ideas, and support for my blog and newsletters and to my agent, Mary Lalli of Westport Entertainment for your belief in my work and your support of my career.

Special thanks to our editor at Rodale, Julie Will, for your clever ideas and mostly for always being there with just the right answers. I am so proud to be working with you. I look forward to many more projects together.

Biggest thanks to *The Biggest Loser* contestants—past and present, onscreen and offscreen. You all have such amazing stories; it has been a gift to know you and to work with each of you. Without you, this book wouldn't have been written. With you, a nation is inspired—thank you!

Melissa Roberson

To my friend and coauthor, Cheryl: If I couldn't whoop it up with you over the phone, I don't know what I'd do! And to my other coauthor, Lisa Wheeler, who is the consummate professional and always a pleasure to work with.

To everyone at Reveille and NBC who makes my work possible, including Chad Bennett, Mark Koops, and Kat Elmore: You always, always help me get the job done.

To my Rodale family, especially editor Julie Will, whom I implicitly trust, and Glenn Abel, who helps make BiggestLoserClub.com possible; also Greg Hottinger and Michael Scholtz, who bring great wisdom and care to members of BiggestLoserClub.com; and Gregg Michaelson, David Krivda, Laura Fields, Robin Shallow, Ellie Prezant, and Sharisse Brutto.

To Sal, who makes the bed and loads *and* empties the dishwasher when I am on deadline.

And to all the cast members of *The Biggest Loser:* Your heart and courage blow me away every single season.

Lisa Wheeler

To my fabulous coauthors, Cheryl Forberg and Melissa Roberson, for their expert knowledge and commitment to health and wellness for all. And especially to Julie Will, our diligent and patient editor at Rodale. I don't know how you pull us and the content all together (magic?). Being part of such a wonderful team makes this work a gift.

To the *Biggest Loser* team! Everyone that I come in contact with at *The Biggest Loser,* NBC, and Reveille feed my creativity and facilitate my success, especially Chad Bennett and Mark Koops. I am constantly inspired by my fellow trainers Bob Harper and Jillian Michaels, whom I have partnered with since the beginning on the workout DVDs. I hope that I can continue to spread their positive message.

I would also like to give a special thanks (and kiss!) to Jessica Davis for her expert eye at the photo shoot for the fitness portion of this book. Not only is she detailed, smart, and funny, but she also makes everyone feel comfortable and pulls out their best.

I could not have written a word of this book without the guidance, inspiration, and encouragement (whether they know it or not) from the following people: Tim Amos, Lashaun Dale, Petra Kolber, Deborah Praver, Cal Pozo, and my dear mother, Helen Wheeler.

And finally, the most important people of all—the *Biggest Loser* contestants. All of you, whether you win, go home, make it to the show, or start your own community programs, inspire the world to make the changes necessary to live healthy vibrant lives.

Index

Underscored page references indicate sidebars and tables. **Boldface** references indicate photographs.

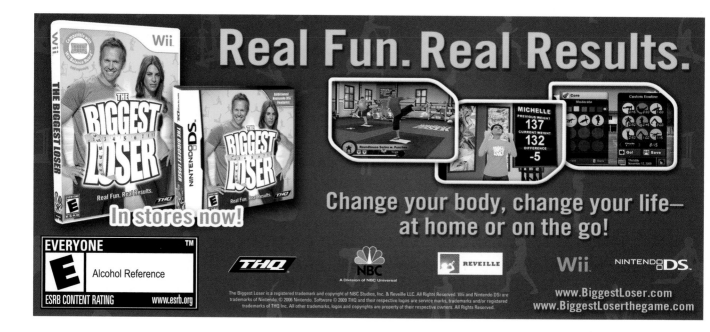

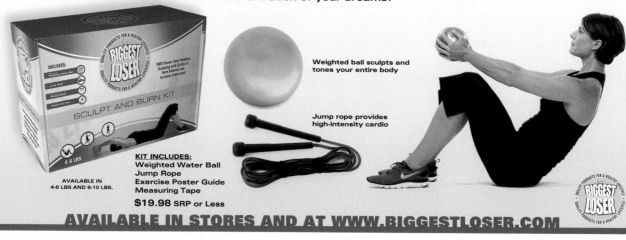

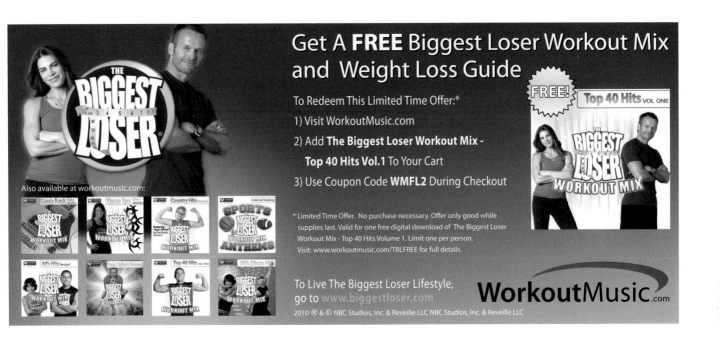
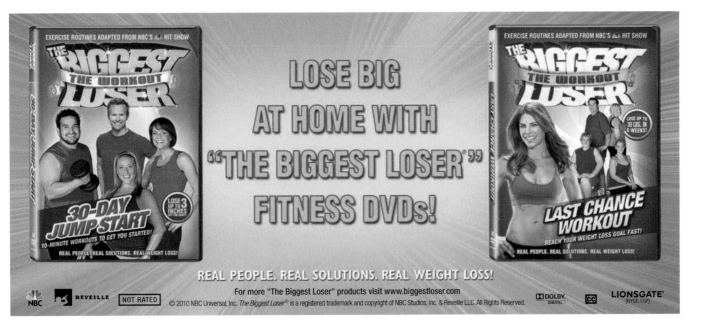

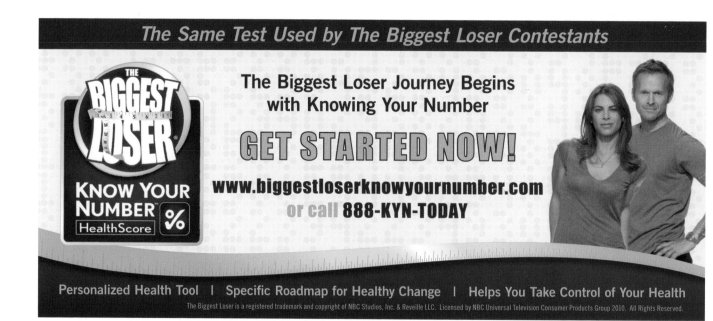
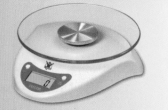
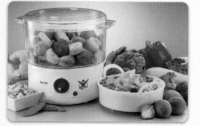
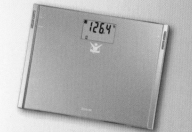

THE BIGGEST LOSER

RESORT

FITNESS RIDGE

FOR FITNESS. FOR FUN. FOR HEALTH. FOR RESULTS. FOR LIFE.

Whatever your focus, our award-winning, compassionate boot camp will give you the results you're aiming for.

biggestloserresort.com | toll free: 888-870-2639 | email: reservations@biggestloserresort.com

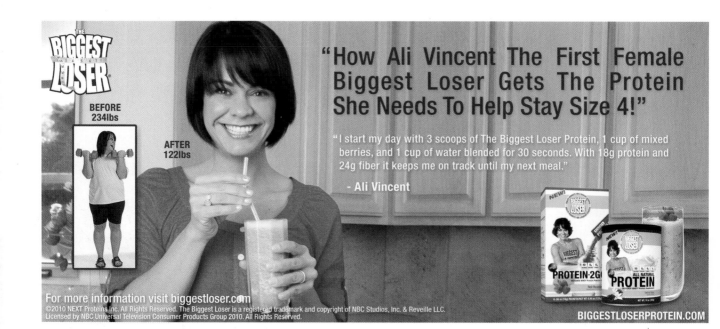

"How Ali Vincent The First Female Biggest Loser Gets The Protein She Needs To Help Stay Size 4!"

"I start my day with 3 scoops of The Biggest Loser Protein, 1 cup of mixed berries, and 1 cup of water blended for 30 seconds. With 18g protein and 24g fiber it keeps me on track until my next meal."

— Ali Vincent

BEFORE 234lbs

AFTER 122lbs

For more information visit biggestloser.com

BIGGESTLOSERPROTEIN.COM

IT'S TIME TO LOSE EVEN MORE WEIGHT

The **bodybugg®** personal calorie management system is the best tool available to help you stay in control of your weight loss. When worn, it tracks how many calories you burn every minute of the day. To live The Biggest Loser lifestyle and for more information about the bodybugg system, go to **www.biggestloser.com**

Used every day by the contestants on NBC's THE BIGGEST LOSER. PC and Mac compatible.

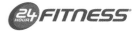

Also available in the *New York Times* best-selling Biggest Loser series...

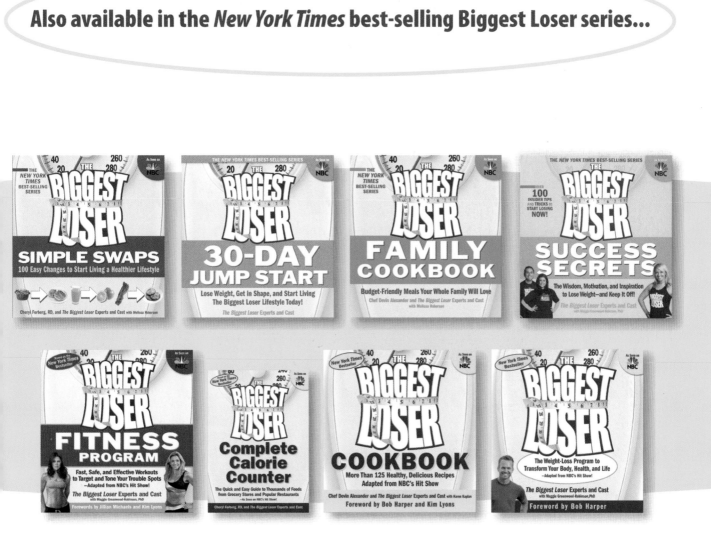

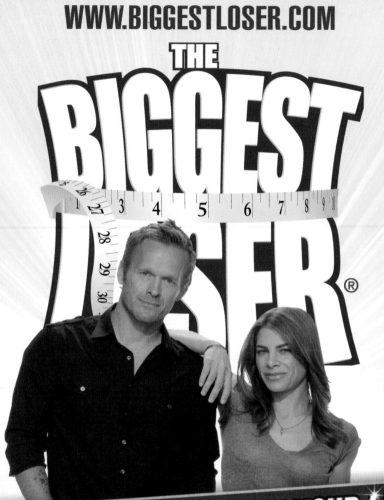